THE
KETOGENIC
& HYPOTOXIC
DIET

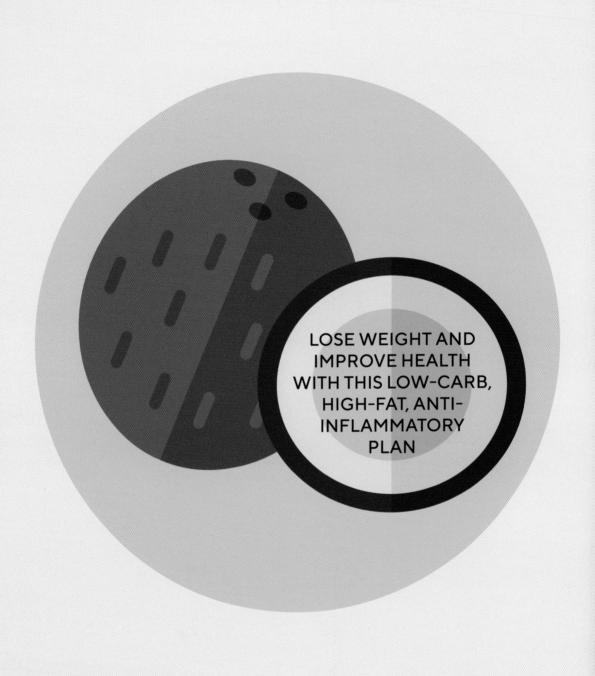

LOSE WEIGHT AND
IMPROVE HEALTH
WITH THIS LOW-CARB,
HIGH-FAT, ANTI-
INFLAMMATORY
PLAN

OLIVIA CHARLET

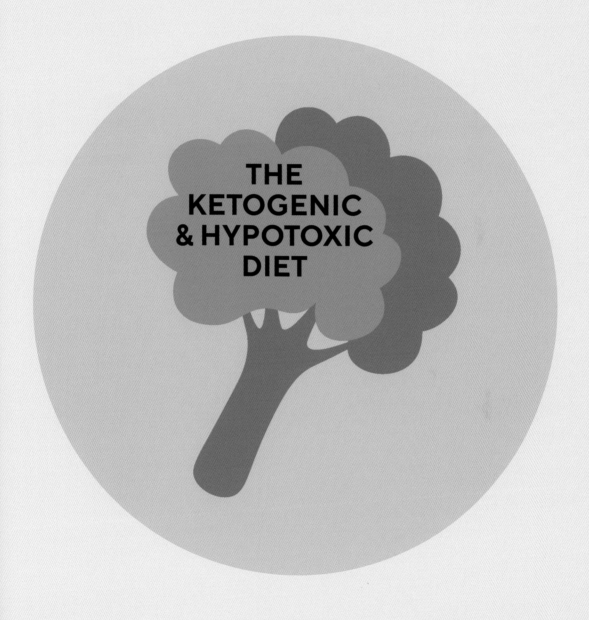

THE KETOGENIC & HYPOTOXIC DIET

eddison
BOOKS LIMITED

This edition published in Great Britain in 2019
by Eddison Books Limited
St Chad's House, 148 King's Cross Road,
London WC1X 9DH
www.eddisonbooks.com

British Library Cataloguing-in-Publication data
available on request.

ISBN 978-1-85906-433-7

10 9 8 7 6 5 4 3 2 1

Printed in China

PLEASE NOTE
It is recommended that you seek professional medical advice
before embarking on any new diet plan. The author and publisher
cannot accept any responsibility for health issues resulting from
the practice of any of the principles, techniques and recipes
included in this book.

CONTENTS

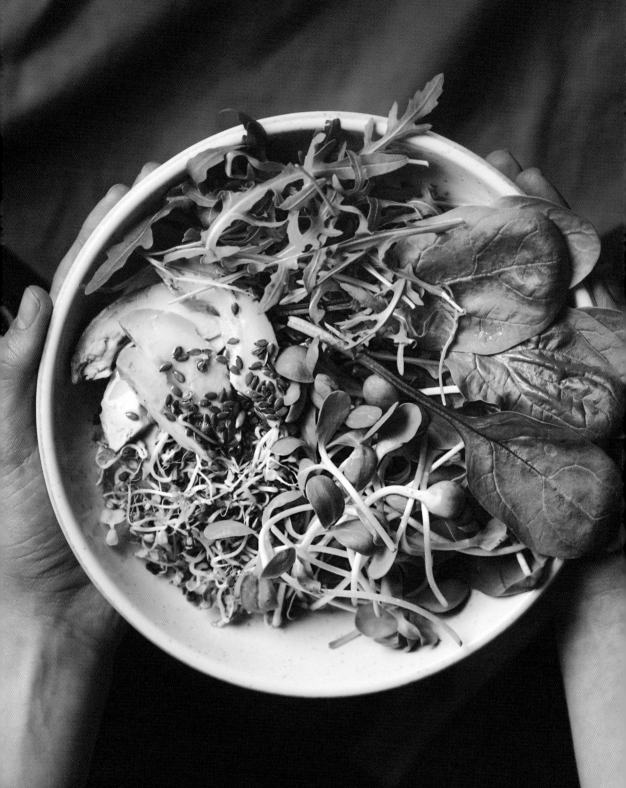

INTRODUCTION

More good fats and (a lot) less sugar of every kind: the ketogenic diet offers **a path to healthier eating and to fighting the many diseases and conditions** that can be linked to modern eating habits, such as obesity, diabetes, inflammatory disorders, autoimmune diseases and cancer.

However, **this doesn't mean you can gorge on meat, cold cuts, cheese, butter or even pesticide-filled vegetables**. Because, when the ketogenic diet isn't followed in an informed way, it can actually be harmful to your health. It's important to consider the current realities of animal farming and industrial agriculture as well as the environment and its impact on your health. It's important, too, to make the right choices to avoid absorbing too many harmful pollutants, chemical products and antibiotics.

Furthermore, some of the key foods in the 'standard' ketogenic diet (such as meat and dairy products) should be avoided – or even completely cut out in the case of most dairy products. These foods are recognized as inflammatory and highly stressful to our digestive tracts, which are already so damaged by modern processed foods. To be beneficial to your health, **the ketogenic diet must therefore also be hypotoxic** – dairy free, gluten free and with only moderate amounts of mostly organic animal protein.

Adopting a ketogenic and hypotoxic diet will often mean a complete upheaval of your dietary habits, and pose a serious challenge to the misconceptions you may have about nutrition. But it's definitely something worth pursuing.

You'll also see that this diet is extremely tasty, rich in authentic flavours and quality products, and a world away from what the food industry offers in supermarkets.

Are you ready for an enjoyable way
to rediscover the true taste of food and
take care of yourself?

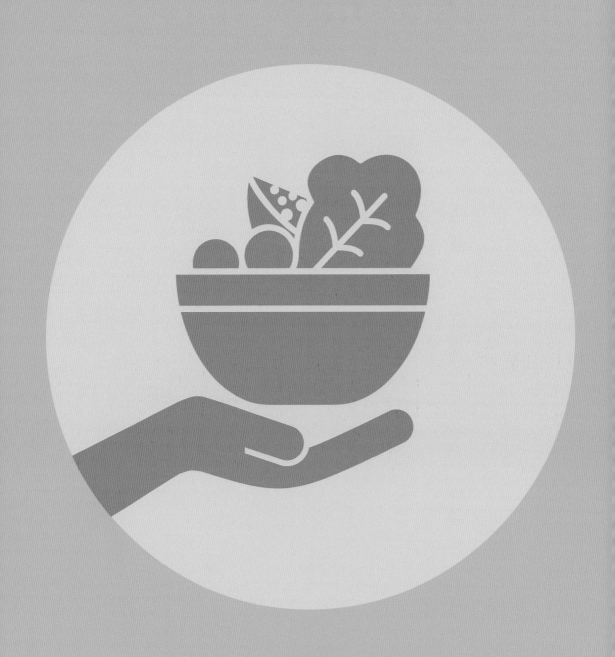

1

WHAT IS THE KETOGENIC & HYPOTOXIC DIET?

A DIFFERENT DISTRIBUTION OF CALORIFIC SUPPLY

The ketogenic diet is a way of eating based on **drastically reducing carbohydrates** (sugars, starches and grains) and where the **calorific supply comes mainly from lipids** (fats).

The diet is based on the latest research in mitochondrial medicine (from 'mitochondria', the energy generators located at the centre of a cell), which highlights the fact that our bodies are not intended to eat so many 'sugars'. The analysis is clear: we currently consume foods we are not genetically designed for, and these foods result in many inflammatory processes.

The distribution of calorific intake in the ketogenic diet runs counter to standard dietary recommendations, in which carbohydrates represent half or more of the calorific intake.

In summary, the ketogenic diet is:
• rich in fats (good fatty acids)
• balanced in proteins (including plant proteins)
• very poor in carbohydrates
It will also provide the vitamins, minerals and phytonutrients your body needs for a number of reactions – in particular, enzymatic reactions.

To clarify, here's a quick reminder of what fats, proteins and carbohydrates are.

FATS

Fats refers to **all fats**. These can derive from animals (butter, cream, cheese, meat) or from plants (seeds, oily fruit, oils). Some fats are called 'essential' as they can come only from food. One example is omega-3 fatty acid – vital to our health but often missing from our meals, leading to inflammatory processes. Fatty acids form the structure of the membrane of every cell. They are also involved in the creation of some hormones and ensure the movement of certain proteins and hormones in the blood. These fatty acids also play a key role in managing inflammatory and allergic phenomena, transmitting signals and activating protein-producing genes.

Within this large family of fats, we need to distinguish between the 'good' and the 'bad' fatty acids, the latter promoting inflammation and leading to a number of diseases. Fatty acids are distinguished by the length of their carbon chain (from four to thirty-two carbons and most often eighteen) and the nature of the bonds (single or double) joining the atoms together. There are two major branches of fatty acids: saturated fatty acids (with no double bonds) and unsaturated fatty acids (with one or more double bonds).

SATURATED FATTY ACIDS

These fatty acids are components of the cell membranes and of fuel specific to certain cell tissues. Some may be required for physical effort. We also need to distinguish between saturated fatty acids from animal sources and those from plant sources. In fact, the presence of excess animal-derived saturated fats is pro-inflammatory, especially when they are nonorganic (containing concentrated foreign chemicals and antibiotic elements) and linked to trans molecules (as in grilled meat cooked inappropriately – see the box on page 12). Unlike animal-based saturated fatty acids, **some plant-based saturated fatty acids contain a significant amount of medium-chain fatty acids (MCFAs) or medium-chain triglycerides (MCTs)**, which have a beneficial effect on our bodies. These MCTs rapidly release MCFAs (essentially octanoic acid, capric acid and lauric acid) into the digestive tract, then pass rapidly into the blood, where they are oxidized to produce compounds called ketones. These ketones replace glucose in supplying energy to the cells. Coconut oil is richest in MCTs, followed by red palm oil and then butter (although, as butter contains casein, a protein that can cause dairy intolerances, it is not indicated within the framework of a hypotoxic ketogenic diet).

The main sources of saturated fatty acids are: meat, cold cuts, bacon, eggs, olives (a mix of saturated and unsaturated fatty acids), cocoa butter, shea butter, nonhydrogenated red palm oil and coconut oil. Dairy products (butter, cream, cheese and milk) are also a main source, though they won't be recommended in this book for reasons that will become clear.

IN A TRADITIONAL DIET
- **Carbohydrates** represent **50 to 55 per cent** of the total energy supply.
- **Fats** represent **35 to 40 per cent** of the total energy supply.
- **Proteins** represent **10 to 15 per cent** of the total energy supply.

IN THE KETOGENIC DIET
- **Carbohydrates** represent **5 to 10 per cent** of the total energy supply.
- **Fats** represent **70 to 80 per cent** (or even more) of the total energy supply.
- **Proteins** represent **15 to 20 per cent** of the total energy supply.

CARBOHYDRATES

FATS

PROTEINS

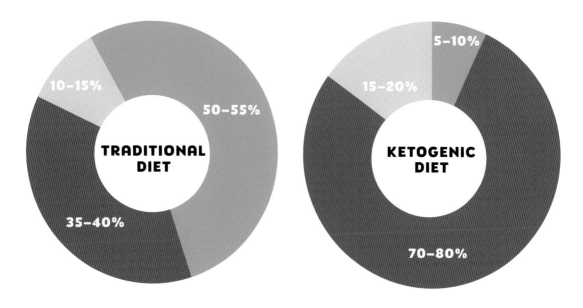

HYDROGENATION, COOKING METHODS AND TRANS FATTY ACIDS

Fatty acids in their natural form have a specific spatial form called 'cis'. Industrial hydrogenation (a process using unsaturated plant oils to make margarine more or less solid at room temperature and able to withstand high cooking temperatures) changes this cis configuration into a 'trans' configuration. These trans fatty acids are considered to be harmful to our health as they increase cardiovascular risks. In fact, our enzymes can no longer recognize or correctly use the processed polyunsaturated fatty acid. There will therefore be less of this in the cell membranes, which will have an enormous impact on the entire cell function, especially in the brain. Cooking certain delicate oils has a similar effect, transforming their configuration to trans. If we heat oil to the point where the polyunsaturated fatty acids start to smoke, we 'break' the oil, creating a toxic substance called acrolein, which is carcinogenic.

The only fats that can be used for cooking, due to their heat resistance, are the following:
- nondeodorized coconut oil
- red palm oil
- cocoa butter
- organic goose fat and duck fat

Please note: Ideally, it's best not to exceed a cooking temperature of 100°C (212°F). Opt for gentle steam cooking, instead, especially using a steam cooker.

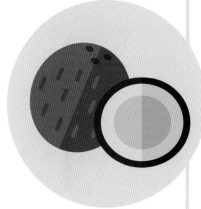

UNSATURATED FATTY ACIDS

These include monounsaturated fatty acids and polyunsaturated fatty acids.

- **Monounsaturated fatty acids** have only one double bond. They are not called 'essential' as they can be synthesized by the body from unsaturated fatty acids. We call them **omega-9s**, the most important of which is **oleic acid**. These fatty acids help to protect the cardiovascular system. **The main sources of monounsaturated fatty acids are:** olives, avocados, macadamia nuts, hazelnuts and, to a lesser extent, almonds. Two animal-based fats – goose fat and duck fat – are also of interest for their omega-9 levels. Semi-solid at room temperature, the fats contain approximately 35 per cent saturated fatty acids, 52 per cent monounsaturated fatty acids (omega-9) and 13 per cent polyunsaturated fatty acids (omega-6 and omega-3). Their levels of omega-3s naturally depend on the foods eaten by the birds (flaxseeds, herbs, or corn or soy flour).

- **Polyunsaturated fatty acids (PUFAs)** or **essential fatty acids (EFAs)** have at least two double bonds, allowing them to play a vital role in many metabolic reactions. The two main examples are **linoleic acid (precursor of omega-6s) and alpha-linolenic acid (precursor of omega-3s)**. We call these 'essential' fatty acids because the body cannot function without them nor can it synthesize them.

- **Omega-3s**, especially eicosapentaenoic acid (EPA) and docosahexaenoic acid (DHA), are used for the synthesis of series-3 prostaglandins (series-3) – substances derived from unsaturated fatty

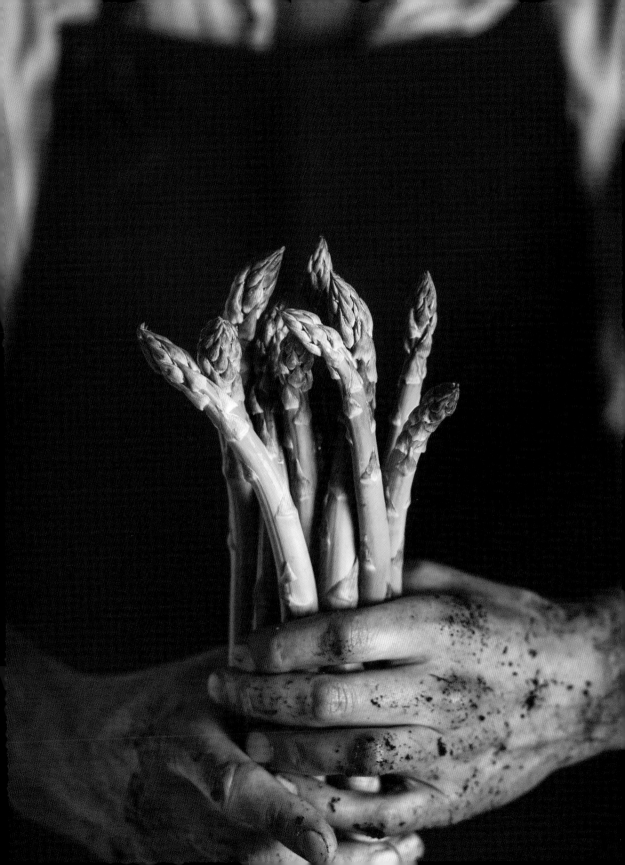

acids that play a cell mediator role. The series-3 prostaglandins reduce and interrupt inflammatory processes. They play an essential role by helping to prevent multiple conditions linked to the onset or maintenance of inflammatory phenomena, such as cardiovascular, allergic and autoimmune diseases, and even some cancers or illnesses linked to brain function. These prostaglandins support the immune system, increase sensitivity to insulin (thereby helping with weight regulation and the prevention of type 2 diabetes), and regulate blood pressure by modifying vascular elasticity and improving skin hydration. **The main sources of omega-3s are:** oily fish, fish oils (directly in the form of EPA and DHA), certain oily fruit, seeds such as flaxseed, chia seeds and sacha inchi seeds, camelina oil, rapeseed oil, sacha inchi oil (in the form of alpha-linolenic acid) and some microalgae (rich in EPA and DHA).

- **Omega-6s** are also vital, but it's important not to take these fatty acids to excess. In fact, many chronic diseases are marked by the overproduction of pro-inflammatory series-2 prostaglandins (as well as other eicosanoids, a larger family of mediators to which prostaglandins belong) made from the omega-6 fatty acid arachidonic acid. Its direct sources include the fattier tissues of meat, dairy products and eggs from hens not fed with flaxseed, while indirect sources include oils such as corn oil, sunflower oil, soy oil and grape seed oil. It's extremely important to ensure the right balance between our intake of omega-3s and our intake of omega-6s to prevent certain types of disease (see the box below). **The main sources of omega-6s are:** some oily fruit and seeds, oils such as corn oil or soy oil, certain kinds of meat (depending on the animals' diet), eggs and processed foods.

WATCH OUT FOR THE OMEGA-3/OMEGA-6 RATIO!

In a diet dominated by processed foods, the consumption of omega-6s is often too high, with an insufficient intake of omega-3s. The general ratio of omega-3s to omega-6s is around 1 to 15, maybe even 1 to 30 (or worse still, 1 to 40 in the United States). This is pro-inflammatory. The norm should be closer to 1 to 4, and indeed for some inflammatory diseases, 1 to 2. Researchers such as Mary Clarke, a PhD student in Nutritional Education at Kansas State University, explain that the ratio of omega-6s to omega-3s was 1 to 1 until the twentieth century. In fact, in the old days, animals ate grass, wild plants and flaxseeds, with the result that their meat naturally contained a significant level of omega-3s. Today, animals are mostly fed on corn or soy flour (often genetically modified). As a result, their meat is too rich in pro-inflammatory omega-6s. This helps the meat-eaters among us to understand the importance of opting for meat from free-range animals fed mainly on fresh plants, by foraging and using ingredients derived from organic agriculture. To restore the proper omega-3/omega-6 balance, it's also important to check the omega-3/omega-6 ratio on the labels of vegetable oils to make sure they are good for your health. Try also to increase your consumption of small oily fish and limit your consumption of ready-made processed foods, which are often high in omega-6 oils.

Conclusion: We shouldn't banish omega-6s entirely as we require those fatty acids as well. All we need is to find the proper omega-3/omega-6 balance. It's worth noting that series-1 prostaglandins, which are synthesized from a specific family of omega-6s (dihomo-gamma-linolenic acid – DGLA – to which oil of evening primrose and borage oil belong), have a beneficial effect on inflammation. They are often given as a food supplement in parallel with EPA and DHA in cases of inflammatory processes.

PROTEINS

These can be **animal-based** (meat, fish, eggs, dairy products) or **plant-based** (pulses, grains, oily fruits and seeds, seaweed). Proteins are found in all living matter as large molecules that provide material for the construction, replacement and repair of our bodies' cells and tissues. Proteins are the building blocks of our bodies: they build our bones, cartilage, muscles, skin and hair. They are composed of chains of elements known as amino acids. Some of these acids, including tryptophan, lysine and methionine, are called 'essential' because our bodies cannot make them on their own.

CARBOHYDRATES

These include **all sugars**: the sugars contained in sweet foods as well as those found in grains (pasta, rice, bread), milk and dairy products, fruit and vegetables. Commonly referred to as 'sugars', these carbohydrates, unlike proteins and fats, are not essential nutrients because our body can make them from other nutrients. This is why we can drastically reduce carbohydrates without fear for our health – and even benefit greatly from such a reduction. This is precisely what the ketogenic diet is all about.

A KETOGENIC AND LOW-CARB DIET

The ketogenic diet is low in carbohydrates. In this sense, it belongs to what are called low-carb diets. Within this group, are:

- **The paleo diet.** This is based on consuming unprocessed natural products (lean meat, fish, vegetables and fruit, seeds) and cutting out grains. The proportion of carbohydrates still makes up approximately 20–40 per cent of the total energy supply. The paleo isn't a low-carb diet but could be considered a first step.
- **The Atkins diet.** This diet recommends greatly restricting carbohydrates at the beginning of the programme and then a gradual reintroduction up to the 'Atkins carbohydrate balance threshold', which is the maximum amount of carbohydrates you can consume without putting on weight, measured at 45–100 g (1½–3½ oz) of carbohydrates per day. Compared to the paleo and Atkins methods, the ketogenic diet goes even further in the restriction of carbohydrates (5–10 per cent of total energy intake), which not only leads to many health benefits but is also less rich in proteins.

THE REAL HARM IN SUGAR & CARBOHYDRATES

ARE CARBOHYDRATES AT THE ROOT OF DISEASES OF MODERN LIFE?

In the ketogenic diet, 'sugars' in their widest sense (carbohydrates) are labelled as enemy number one. Our eating habits have largely evolved towards carbohydrates, which have become ubiquitous in our meals: ever more grains and starches, sugars and sugar-based products, and processed foods with refined sugar. In the UK, all age groups consume more than double the officially recommended maximum of 5 per cent of total energy intake through 'free' sugars, which are sugars added to products or found in honey, syrup or fruit juices. This is a real public health problem, which, contrary to popular belief, is nothing new. Studies carried out on Egyptian mummies show, for example, that the introduction of grains into the Ancient Egyptian diet coincided with an increase in tooth cavities, cardiovascular diseases and obesity!

It's no coincidence that obesity and type 2 diabetes have become truly epidemic in the West today. **It's becoming increasingly clear that there's a link between the overconsumption of carbohydrates and the diseases of modern life as well as neurodegenerative and autoimmune diseases, cancer, and inflammatory and cardiovascular diseases.** At the same time, there are more and more scientific studies demonstrating the benefit of reducing carbohydrate consumption to prevent these diseases (in particular cardiovascular diseases and cancers), as well as to lose weight.

So why do the health authorities continue to advise us to eat so many carbohydrates, as well as recommending for the most part that we consume grains at every meal? This is simply down to the power of the sugar and grain industries! They even succeeded in influencing some significant studies that turned our attention towards another supposed enemy – fats. This led to fats being blamed for all the

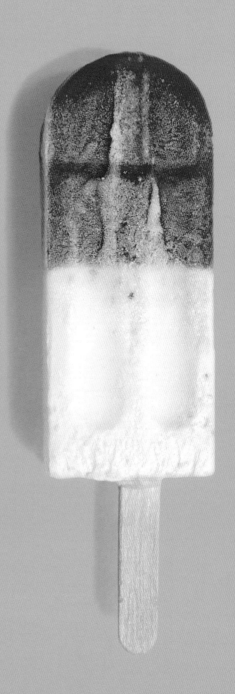

harm for which sugars were in fact responsible. Many nutritional recommendations have been based on this enormous lie, resulting in most consumers today believing mistakenly that in order to eat healthily without gaining weight, they need to reduce their consumption of fats. Ever since the health authorities in the United States started to recommend in the 1950s that people eat less fat, but have grains at every meal, the obesity rate has increased steadily. Fortunately, things are beginning to change.

METABOLISM OF CARBOHYDRATES VS METABOLISM OF FATS

To clearly understand why an excess of carbohydrates is harmful to our bodies, it's important to understand exactly how they are assimilated, and then compare this with the metabolism of fats (the main source of energy in a ketogenic diet).

The metabolism of carbohydrates: carbohydrates ingested in the body are transformed into glucose, also called blood sugar. This is broken down and converted into energy – known as cellular respiration. The blood sugar level is regulated by insulin, a hormone produced in the pancreas, whose role it is to release sugar into the cells to help them function. The insulin receptors are like locks on a door, with the insulin acting as the key, thus allowing the sugar to enter into the cells so that they can be used by the mitochondria to produce the energy carrier adenosine triphosphate (ATP). The unused glucose is then stored either in the liver (hepatic glycogen) or in the muscles (muscle glycogen), or, when these reserves become full, in the form of triglycerides (fats) in the fat tissue. What happens when we consume too many carbohydrates? The pancreas has to produce even more insulin, and the insulin receptors in the cellular membrane become saturated. They no longer allow glucose to properly enter into the cells to be used by the mitochondria, the energy centres that produce the ATP, meaning very little glucose manages to get into the cell.

The sugar then accumulates to dangerous levels in the blood, and the pancreas tries to produce more and more insulin to release into the cells – a phenomenon known as insulin resistance. This excess sugar stagnates to a certain extent in the blood, and a large amount is also stored in the fat tissue. Chronically high insulin levels can lead to acne, excess weight, type 2 diabetes, inflammation, cardiovascular diseases, hypertension, cystic ovarian syndrome and cancer.

The metabolism of fats: this is controlled by the liver, which transforms one part into energy (energy output into the mitochondria by beta-oxidation) and the other part into steroid hormones (from the cholesterol). The liver also helps to produce eicosanoids, which are involved in all the vital balances of our bodies (such as heart rate, blood pressure, inflammation, vasoconstriction and regulating gastric secretions), and subtly regulates gene expression.

What happens when we consume too few carbohydrates, perhaps even almost none, and lots of fats (the ketogenic diet)? In this situation, the liver uses fats as the main source of energy. To do this, it transforms them into ketones or ketone bodies: acetoacetate, beta-hydroxybutyrate (BHB) and acetone. The process takes place at the level of the hepatic mitochondria, which are then stimulated to produce ketone bodies from the Acetyl-CoA molecule. These bodies then pass into the blood, which is then the state of nutritional ketosis (see also page 27).

The same phenomenon is produced during prolonged fasting. **Ketone bodies are the ideal fuel for our cells**, including our heart and brain cells as well as the muscles and the renal cortex. The liver uses ketone bodies to produce the fuel required for the proper functioning of our bodies. The mitochondria thus function with a completely different metabolism, which, as we will see later on in this book, proves to be especially beneficial for our health on various levels.

SO WHAT DOES HYPOTOXIC MEAN?

It's often assumed that the ketogenic diet involves a high consumption of fatty meat and full-fat dairy products, such as butter, cheese and cream. In fact, to be beneficial for our health, a ketogenic diet has to be hypotoxic.

Fatty meat and full-fat dairy are major sources of toxins and are pro-inflammatory, with fats high in arachidonic acid, trans fats (as in pro-oxidant grilled meat), casein (in cheese, for example, which has a detrimental effect on the intestinal lining), leucine and antibiotics. So it's impossible for these foods to be beneficial for our health.

It's important therefore to adopt a ketogenic diet that is fundamentally hypotoxic. This aspect of the diet is vital for our health. Say yes to fats – but not to just any kind!

The three main principles of the ketogenic and hypotoxic diet are as follows:

PROTEINS, CAREFULLY CHOSEN AND MODERATELY CONSUMED

All toxins, such as pollutants, heavy metals, antibiotic residues and pesticides, accumulate in animal fats. This is why it's vital to choose good-quality meat from animals raised organically and fed on grass – not on grains high in pro-inflammatory omega-6s). You can even opt for a vegetarian or vegan diet when following the principles of a hypotoxic ketogenic diet (see 'Recipes', starting on page 104).

Furthermore, animal meats are acidifying, even when the quality is good. They contribute to the acidifying of the body when consumed in excess and without a large helping of green vegetables. They are also a source of pro-inflammatory components, including arachidonic acid, leucine and pro-oxidant iron. Moreover, when cooked to high temperatures (on a grill or barbecue, for instance), animal meats produce carcinogenic substances, as well as 'glycation end products', which accelerate aging and tissue oxidation. For all these

reasons, meat should be consumed in moderation. It may even be cut out completely, if you prepare meals instead that are properly balanced in plant proteins – a simple thing to do.

Also, since animal fats accumulate heavy metals, it's important to opt for small oily fish, such as anchovies or sardines, over large ones, such as tuna and salmon, which, because they have eaten the small ones, are even more concentrated in heavy metals. The heavy metal mercury, for example, is a powerful neurotoxin found in varying quantities in most fish.

NO DAIRY PRODUCTS OR GLUTEN

Cheese, butter, cream and even yogurt contain lactose and galactose, which, when consumed in excess, accumulate in body tissues, in particular in the lens (causing opacification of the lens and risk of cataract) and the nerve sheath (carrying a risk of neuropathy). Another major toxin found in dairy products, even more detrimental to our health, is casein, which disrupts the central nervous system by producing opioid substances and makes the intestinal lining more porous. The consequences of this include concentration problems, mood swings, chronic fatigue, irritable bowels, food intolerance, skin problems, ear, nose and throat problems, and migraines – not forgetting a weakening and disruption of the immune defences.

Not only that, but dairy products are also pro-inflammatory. They contain hormones and growth promoters, suspected of causing certain cancers and autoimmune diseases (in particular, but not limited to, type 1 diabetes and Hashimoto's thyroiditis), and inflammatory and neurodegenerative diseases.

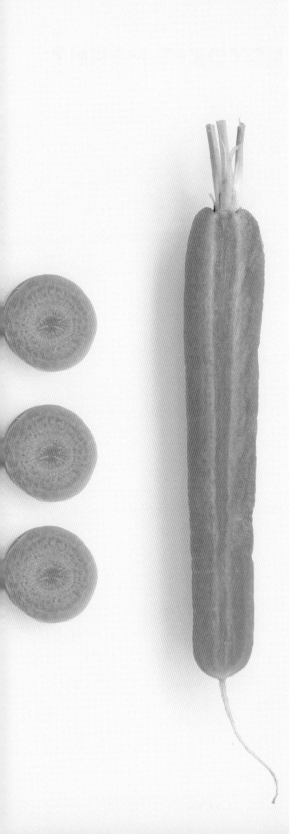

The ketogenic diet is naturally low in gluten as it excludes grains, pseudo-grains and processed foods (which often contain gluten in the form of additives). Gluten, like casein, acts on the brain receptors with effects similar to opiate drugs, leading to mood swings and an addiction to products containing it. Gluten also belongs to the large group of 'prolamins', which constantly attack our intestinal lining. We now understand the importance of keeping this lining healthy due to its crucial role in the development of many diseases.

A MOSTLY ORGANIC DIET

As stated already, when it comes to meat, it's best to choose organic. But this isn't enough. For obvious health reasons, it's always preferable to choose plant foods grown in living soil, rich in microorganisms and without added chemicals. In the medium and long terms, and depending on the state of our internal detoxification system, putting chemical and toxic substances into our bodies could have serious consequences on our health and fertility, and impact future generations.

On top of this, organic vegetables are nutritionally much richer in vitamins and minerals and, above all, contain many phytonutrients and powerful anticarcinogens. It's time to make the right choices for your health and our planet!

WHAT TO EAT
& WHAT TO AVOID

The ketogenic and hypotoxic diet is based on the following food groups, which are covered in greater detail in the chapter 'Key foods' – starting on page 30.

KETOGENIC KEY FOODS

Fats: mainly organic oils rich in omega-3s and in medium-chain triglycerides (MCTs), including camelina oil, rapeseed oil, coconut oil, red palm oil, cocoa butter and good-quality animal fats such as duck fat

Oily fruit and seeds: almonds, walnuts, chia seeds and flaxseeds, for example

Good-quality meat and poultry: organic and free-range

Small oily fish: especially anchovies and sardines

Algae: especially seaweed, spirulina and klamath

Eggs

Some low-carbohydrate vegetables

Some fruit: olives, avocado, coconut and berries, for example

Herbs, spices and vinegars: especially turmeric and ginger

Some 'super foods': including acerola, spirulina, raw cacao and sprouted grains

Some specific sweet foods: such as coconut sugar and kitul, yacon and carob syrups – in moderation and as part of a low-carb diet

THE KETOGENIC DIET AVOIDS:

Sugar and all sugar products: including honey, jam, sweets, white sugar and cane sugar

All processed foods: including biscuits, pastries and convenience foods

Grains and leguminous plants: unless gluten free and in moderation in their sprouted form

Vegetables rich in carbohydrates and most fruit

All dairy products: including yogurt, butter, cream and chees. These are excluded mainly because they are pro-inflammatory. In fact, all dairy products, even plain yogurt, strongly affect insulin response because of the type of sugar they contain.

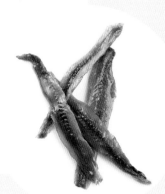

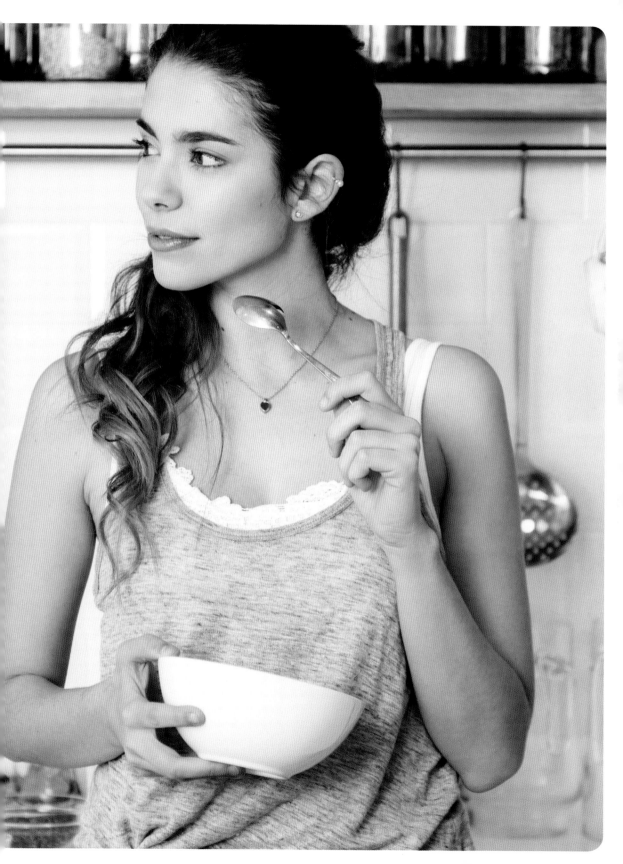

THE BENEFITS

Follow the ketogenic and hypotoxic diet and you can help to prevent and treat certain diseases and dysfunctions.

• If **epilepsy** is at the top of the list of diseases, this is because the ketogenic diet was first used for medical purposes at the very beginning of the twentieth century to treat children with epilepsy who were unresponsive to treatment. In France, for instance, the ketogenic diet has long been associated with epilepsy and is offered in many hospitals providing medical care for children with this disease. In the early 1920s, the American physician Dr Russell Wilder scientifically demonstrated the benefits of this type of nutrition for **people with epilepsy**. He found that the ketone bodies produced by the liver reduced convulsions thanks to the production of the neurotransmitter gamma-aminobutyric acid (GABA), which protected the brain. He therefore developed a strict diet that proved to be highly effective. The arrival of antiepileptic medicines in the 1950s was a game-changer and the diet was gradually abandoned. In the 1990s, Wilder's diet came back into fashion for treating children who were unresponsive to conventional medical treatment (some 30 per cent of cases). Another advantage highlighted was how quickly this beneficial effect manifested itself – from only several days to several weeks after the adoption of a strict ketogenic diet.

• A ketogenic diet can help prevent **type 2 diabetes**, especially for people with a family history of the disease. This is in fact a disease of the metabolism of carbohydrates: the overconsumption of sugar creates insulin resistance. The blood sugar level is no longer being controlled. It becomes chronically too elevated because the insulin receptors in every cell are no longer effective and then become 'resistant' to insulin. As a result, sugar cannot enter the cells and reaches dangerous levels in the blood. This then depletes the pancreas. By drastically reducing sugar intake, the insulin receptors are a lot less called upon, especially in a ketogenic diet rich in omega-3s, allowing these receptors to regain their effectiveness. The ketogenic diet can also be used as a treatment for people with type 2 diabetes, preventing complications that affect the eyes, kidneys, liver and heart, and helping to restore the effectiveness of the insulin receptors.

• The ketogenic diet is also a promising route to treating **Alzheimer's disease**. Scientists are increasingly linking the disease to diabetes, even calling it 'type 3 diabetes' or 'brain diabetes'. Alzheimer's is a neurodegeneration of the brain, where the brain isn't able to correctly use glucose, its usual source of energy. As with 'classic' diabetes, the cells – neural in this case – show a resistance to insulin, preventing sugar from passing through their membrane and therefore from being used. This insulin resistance promotes the forming of senile plaques in the brain, so the brain functions in slow motion, causing memory disorders. But, what if the brain were supplied with another source of energy, namely ketones, derived from fat transformation?

• In general, the ketogenic diet is believed to have positive effects on the brain, and therefore on the prevention and treatment of brain disorders. A number of these disorders have been linked to a diet too high in carbohydrates and deficient in good fats. Dr David Perlmutter, an American neurologist, began working on this issue after his father was diagnosed with **Parkinson's disease**. In his book *Grain Brain*, Dr Perlmutter clearly explains the damaging effects of pro-inflammatory carbohydrates, grains with gluten and dairy products on the brain. He confirms that the consumption of gluten and a diet high in carbohydrates count as among the most important stimulants of inflammatory paths affecting the

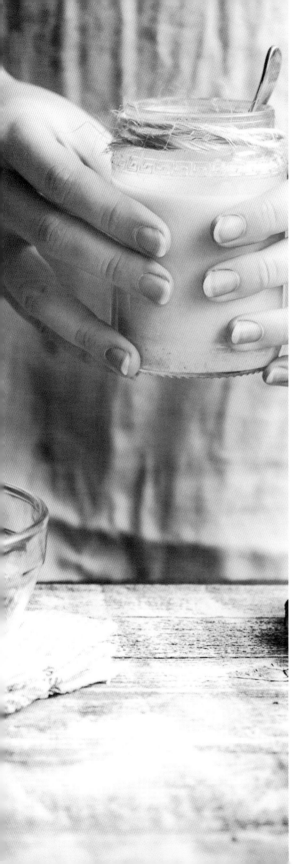

brain. Contrary to popular belief, glucose is not the brain's preferred fuel. In fact, the bonding of sugar molecules to protein molecules in the brain (a phenomenon known as glycation) brings about a shrinking of the brain tissue. Ketone bodies are therefore much healthier for our brains!

• An increasing number of studies are putting forward the benefits of a ketogenic diet for **the prevention and treatment of cancer** as a complement to the patient's treatment. Cancer cells need sugar to grow – it's their one and only fuel. In cancer cells, the mitochondria, the small energy centres, stop working properly. Instead of burning glucose, the cell fills up and expands, promoting tumour growth. By depriving our body of sugar, the development of tumours can be slowed down. This helps to normalize our metabolism and restore a cell's normal functioning. This, in simplified terms, is the link that exists between carbohydrates and cancer.

• The ketogenic diet is also an extremely effective solution for **combating obesity and excess weight**, conditions that are affecting more and more people, in all age groups and across much of the world. We know today that it's excess carbohydrates that are fattening, not excess fats. In fact, when taken in quantities beyond what our body needs, these carbohydrates are stored in our fat tissue in the form of triglycerides, which lead to fat mass gain. An overproduction of insulin, together with a diet high in sugar (both fast and slow) will increase the storage of fatty acids in the fat tissue. By drastically reducing the intake of carbohydrates, we can prevent fat storage.

The ketogenic diet also proves to be an effective solution for controlling the appetite and therefore for eating less. In fact, fats and proteins, largely present in this type of diet, are more satiating than carbohydrates, mainly because they are slower to digest. They also don't present the problem of contributing to the sensation of hunger that is specific to carbohydrates.

• The ketogenic diet also appears to be effective in **the prevention and treatment of cardiovascular diseases**. For decades, these diseases have been associated with the consumption of fats, and there is still a long way to go to disassociate the consumption of fats from high cholesterol and cardiovascular disorders in the minds of a large part of the population. The ketogenic diet has a positive effect on a great number of recognized cardiovascular disease risk factors, especially diabetes and obesity. In addition, because of its high omega-3 content, the diet helps to raise levels of good cholesterol, recognized for its protective benefits on the cardiovascular system.

• The ketogenic diet offers many **benefits for the treatment of inflammatory diseases**, most of which are due to a diet too rich in carbohydrates and deficient in good fats (omega-3s). One of the ketone bodies created by the liver when the body is in ketosis – beta-hydroxybutyrate (BHB) – has an anti-inflammatory effect. This acts on the inflammatory factor involved in the onset of many diseases, such as asthma, osteoarthritis, rheumatism and autoimmune diseases. Researchers at the Yale School of Medicine have demonstrated that BHB blocks inflammatory diseases by inhibiting the inflammasome NLRP3. The body produces BHB during intensive exercise, when on a ketogenic diet and when on a strict or intermittent fast (around 15 hours of fasting).

Additionally, the ketogenic diet increases production of the principal antioxidant naturally secreted by the liver (glutathione) and increases the effectiveness of our energy centres, the mitochondria. More generally, the ketogenic diet allows you to consume more molecules with recognized anti-inflammatory effects, especially omega-3s, which are essential for the production of anti-inflammatory pseudo-hormones known as type 3 prostaglandins (found especially in small oily fish, some microalgae, certain plant-based oils, and some oily fruit and seeds).

The ketogenic diet excludes all pro-inflammatory grains – rich in inflammatory

GLUTEN AND INFLAMMATION: DANGEROUS LIAISONS

Gluten is one of the additives most commonly used by the food and cosmetics industries. It provokes an immune response, causing inflammation, and is responsible for intestinal permeability and intestinal dysbiosis (an imbalance in the microbiota or intestinal flora). This is called intestinal hyperpermeability (or leaky gut syndrome). In this situation, the intestinal barrier no longer plays its role of watchdog and allows entry into the blood of peptides (badly divided chains of amino acids), toxic substances, toxins and pathogenic microorganisms, keeping our immune systems in a constant state of alertness. Casein, the protein in dairy products, produces similar effects.

Two peptides have been identified as 'gluteomorphins' (from gluten) and 'casomorphins'* (from casein). They can be detected with a urine test. The passage into the blood–brain barrier of these peptides (known as 'opioid peptides') disrupts the brain's entire behaviour. The inflammatory stress of the blood–brain barrier due to an alteration in the intestinal lining allows entry into the brain of pathogenic mediators from the digestive tract, opioid peptides from gluten and dairy products that counter the endorphins and lead to states of malaise, behavioural disorders and autoimmune and neurodegenerative diseases.

* Gluteomorphins and casomorphins were identified in the works of Professor Karl Reichelt, doctor in neurochemistry and researcher at the University of Oslo. He published more than 200 scientific articles and has received the university's Snøkloas medical prize for his research studies.

substances, notably prolamins, which include the infamous 'gluten'. Note that corn and millet, and not just wheat, contain gluten, which most food packaging does not currently state. Of the prolamins, the most toxic are alpha-gliadin (wheat), secalin (rye) and hordein (barley), followed by zein (corn).

• Cutting out gluten, drastically reducing carbohydrates, eliminating dairy products and increasing the intake of omega-3s (in particular docosahexaenoic acid – DHA – which plays an important role for the brain) also have a very positive effect on **autistic disorders**. Aspects of these disorders may be explained by the passage of peptides into the blood (which provokes an immune response), by chronic inflammation and by a disruption of the immune system. In a more general sense, this may also explain other disorders such as mood disorders, depression, behavioural disorders, migraine and hyperactivity.

The opioid peptides gluteomorphins and casomorphins (from gluten and dairy products, respectively) – see box opposite – act on the brain's opioid receptors and imitate the effects of opioid drugs such as heroin or morphine. In particular, they target certain areas of the brain such as the temporal lobes, which play a major role in language development and listening comprehension. For people who cannot properly digest gluten or casein, fragments of proteins are absorbed into the body, where they attach themselves to the opioid receptors, changing behaviour as well as certain physiological responses.

• The ketogenic diet may also be used to treat **migraine**. The very first studies on this subject were carried out in the 1920s. These results were confirmed by more recent studies, showing that following the diet reduces the frequency of attacks. This effectiveness is linked to ketones, which have a recognized anti-inflammatory effect. For more than a decade, Dr Marios Hadjivassiliou, Professor of Neurology at the University of Sheffield, has continued to demonstrate that a diet without gluten and low in carbohydrates, which the

ketogenic diet happens to be, can result in the complete disappearance of headaches in patients suffering from gluten intolerance. Casomorphins are also implicated in the causes of migraines, so it can also be important for some sufferers to cut out dairy products. Migraine is also very often linked to a problem of intestinal inflammation.

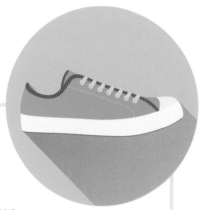

INCREASING ATHLETIC PERFORMANCE

In the 1960s, athletes were advised to favour carbohydrates in order to improve athletic performance and reload glycogen reserves in their muscles, with a ratio of 55 per cent or even 60 per cent carbohydrates for endurance athletes. However, more recent studies go against this practice for improving performance, seeing in it digestive problems due to sugars and inflammation of the intestinal wall due to intensive athletic activity. This creates a fundamental shift in the world of sports! Adopting a ketogenic diet (where the proportion of carbohydrates does not exceed 5–7 per cent of energy intake) helps athletes to improve their insulin sensitivity, reduce oxidative stress, reduce low-grade inflammation that follows athletic activity and improve cellular energy efficiency. The ketone bodies ensure the controlled use of energy substrates by the muscles.

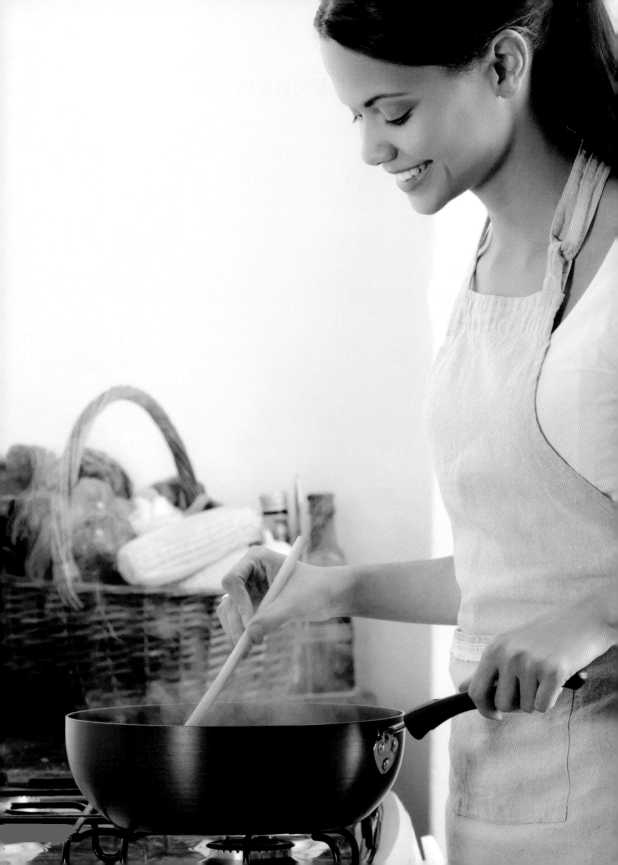

ENJOYING THE BENEFITS

THE SWITCH TO KETOSIS

Simply directing your diet towards fats while also including some protein and very little sugar isn't quite enough to enjoy the many benefits of the ketogenic diet. In fact, the distinctiveness of this way of eating – and its goal – is to make the body switch to another form of functioning or metabolism. In other words, when you follow the diet, the body no longer gets its energy from sugar (via glycolysis and mitochondrial respiration) but from making ketone bodies. This is what is called ketosis.

To make the body switch to ketosis, there are **three key conditions**:
- A drastic restriction in carbohydrate consumption
- A sufficient consumption of fats
- A moderate consumption of protein

However, the maximum threshold of carbohydrates required to switch to ketosis is different for every person. On average, this tends to be less than 50 g (1¾ oz) of carbohydrates per day. Note that this actually means 50 g (1¾ oz) of 'carbohydrates' and not sugar. For some people, who are particularly sedentary, the maximum threshold of carbohydrates will be even lower, around 30 g (1 oz) of carbohydrates per day.

For more active people, the maximum threshold of carbohydrates required to switch to ketosis could be a little higher. In fact, for high-performance athletes, this threshold could be as high as 100 g (3½ oz) of carbohydrates per day. This difference is explained by the much greater number of mitochondria in high-performance athletes.

Your body could take up to three days to switch to ketosis, starting from when you adopt a strictly ketogenic diet and dependent on a few other conditions, such as already being on a diet very low in carbohydrates for several weeks previously. If you simply limit carbohydrates and increase your consumption of good fatty acids (without adopting a strict ketogenic diet), the switch to ketosis could take many weeks, or maybe not happen at all if your carbohydrate levels are still too high, and especially if you are sedentary.

There is a trick to accelerating this process: begin with a fast (a liquid fast with only water and herbal teas) for at least one day, or even two to three days. Follow this fast and your body will rapidly move to ketosis. You can then remain in ketosis by restricting your consumption of carbohydrates to less than 20 g (¾ oz) of carbohydrates per day. You could also choose to do an intermittent fast (a liquid fast from 9 pm to 1 pm the following day) over three days, which is less restricting.

To check that the switch to ketosis has actually taken place, you can perform a urine test (such as Ketostix® or Keto-Diastix®) available from a pharmacy. The tests have the advantage of being easy and quick to use but are not necessarily reliable because they measure the ketones eliminated in the urine and not their concentration in the blood. With such a test, the switch to ketosis is effective when the quantity of ketones is around 15 mg/dl. These urine tests are an inexpensive way to start off on a ketogenic diet for most people, unless you're adopting this way of eating to treat a health issue. In that case, you'll need a more precise measurement, from a blood glucose and blood ketone meter. The various devices available include Precision Xtra® (Abbott), Freestyle Optium Neo® (Abbott) and Nova Max Plus® (Nova). Feel free to talk about these with your doctor. You can also ask for a laboratory blood test (with a prescription).

DOES THE KETOGENIC DIET HAVE ANY SIDE-EFFECTS?

The switch to ketosis – a transition from one metabolism to another – can sometimes be accompanied by a little discomfort, but fortunately only for a short time. These side-effects could include light headache, fatigue, nausea and occasionally constipation if you do not properly follow the main guidelines of the ketogenic diet. Any discomfort manifests itself mainly in the first two to four days. It's often related to dehydration because of the ketogenic diet's diuretic effect (meaning you eliminate more water).

Any incidences of **light headaches, dizziness or fatigue** are linked to dehydration and to mineral deficiency. If this happens, all you need to do is rehydrate well and take in more electrolytes (minerals) for the symptoms to rapidly disappear. Take care with your water intake and drink at least 1.5 litres (3 pints) per day of lightly mineralized spring water, which will hydrate your cells and not have the laxative and therefore demineralizing effect of mineral waters. Also watch your intake of minerals, especially potassium (in avocados, dried herbs, almonds and coconut), calcium (in sardines, almonds, sesame seeds, chia seeds, cabbage and green vegetables), selenium (in brazil nuts and coconut flour) and magnesium (in raw cacao and hazelnuts). You could also include dried seaweed or seaweed tartare in your daily diet. Both are rich in minerals but also very alkaline and high in electrolytes, so it's alright to overeat them! You could also add a little unpasteurized rice miso into your soups to supply probiotics, as well as sodium and electrolytes.

You may also experience **constipation** because of the change in diet and if you don't eat plenty of fibre-rich green vegetables. To prevent this from happening, don't forget to consume a sufficient amount of vegetables (low in carbohydrates). You might also consider seeds (such as psyllium, flax or chia) and fibre-rich coconut flour. Make sure you stay well hydrated, drinking lightly mineralized spring water (mountain spring water). Finally, don't forget to stay active and, in particular, to walk briskly for at least 30 minutes per day, and ideally for at least one hour. Physical exercise is key in promoting good bowel movements and a state of ketosis.

IS THE KETOGENIC DIET FOR EVERYONE?

Everyone, whether in good health or suffering from ill health, should limit their intake of carbohydrate and favour fats in their diet. In practice, this can be done in various ways, depending on your goals, needs or lifestyle. That is why this book offers three ketogenic programmes: weight loss, anti-inflammatory and vegetarian/vegan (see pages 80–103). What matters is that you advance gradually but in a sustainable way towards better and healthier eating habits, and at your own pace.

The ketogenic diet is a way of eating that can be suitable, therefore, for anyone. However, a few precautions must be taken in particular cases.

- **If you suffer from an inflammatory or autoimmune disease, or cancer**, adopting a strict ketogenic diet is essential in order to get results. Don't hesitate to seek support from a specialist for this type of diet. This is bound to involve a more or less extended low-carb stage, depending on your dietary history. It's probably best to go in stages.
- **If you're diabetic** and you wish to adopt a ketogenic diet, talk to your doctor, as it may be necessary to adjust and reduce your treatment over time.
- If you suffer from **renal failure**, don't start a ketogenic diet without the advice of your doctor, as this type of diet is diuretic. In this case, adopting a less restrictive low-carb diet or a paleo diet may be preferable. Short periods of a ketogenic diet may then be integrated – and always, of course, under medical and nutritional supervision.
- **If you suffer from gout or lithiasis**, the same advice applies: try another, less restrictive low-carb alternative.
- **If you are pregnant**, you should not start this type of diet. However, a low-carb diet will be very healthy in this context, and you could start on a ketogenic diet after delivery.

If you have the slightest doubt, or if you require guidance during this change in diet, don't hesitate to consult a ketogenic diet specialist.

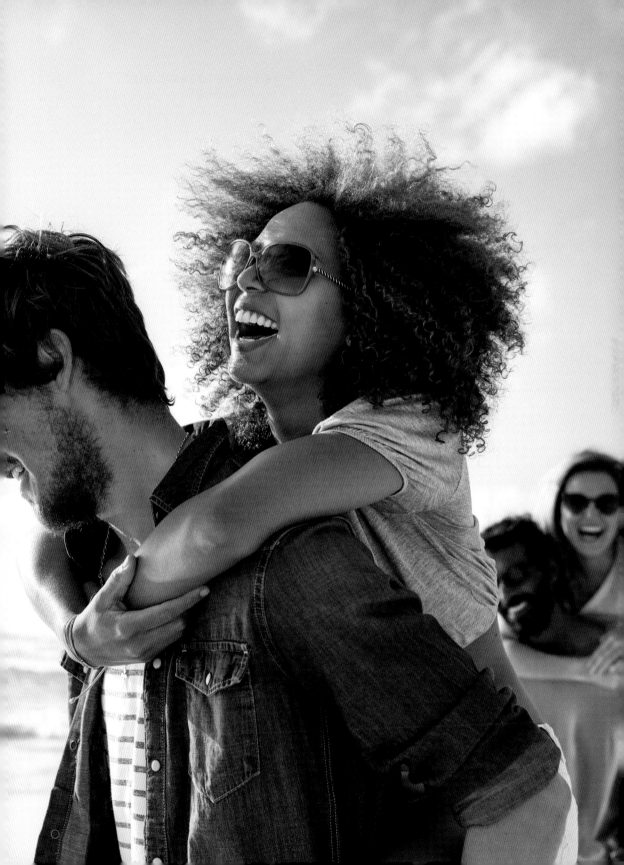

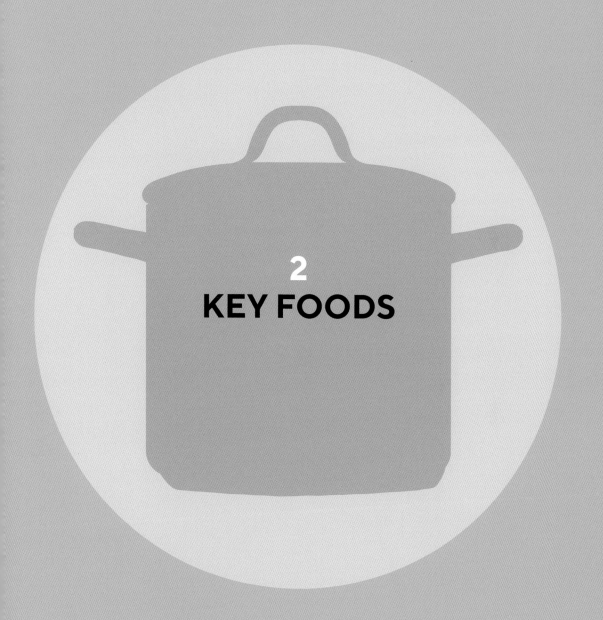

2
KEY FOODS

COCONUT OIL
THE KETOGENIC DIET'S KEY FAT

The distinctive characteristic of cococut oil is its concentration of saturated fatty acids and, in particular, medium-chain triglycerides, or MCTs. These fatty acids help to speed up the transition to ketosis by allowing the liver to naturally produce more ketones per calorie than any other fatty acid.

Ketosis occurs when the body does not have enough glucose for energy, and burns stored fats instead, resulting in the production of ketones within the body. It's a normal metabolic process, caused by a significantly lowered intake of carbs.

Coconut oil is the best source of MCTs, which make up 60 per cent of its fatty acids. Around 45 per cent of this consists of lauric acid, a fatty acid that converts to monolaurin in the body, a compound also found in breast milk. Its purpose is to strengthen a baby's immune system, promote normal brain development and contribute to bone development. In addition, monoluarin has antimicrobial properties – in other words, it can kill bacteria and pathogenic viruses.

WHEN IT COMES TO CHOOSING OIL:

Always opt for a nondeodorized, extra-virgin coconut oil derived from organic farming. This type is generally easy to find in organic stores. Don't go for refined and deodorized oil!

HOW TO USE COCONUT OIL
- In salad dressings
- For cooking meat, fish and vegetables (the oil can withstand high temperatures)
- In pastries (pancakes, crepes, cakes)
- In hot drinks (tea, coffee, maté, hot chocolate), to increase your intake of good fats – just add 1 tablespoon and stir in.

PLEASE NOTE!
Coconut oil is solid below 25°C (77°F) and liquid above this temperature. The transition from one state to the other does not affect its nutritional properties. Store it at room temperature.

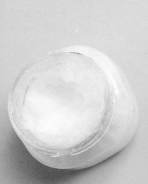
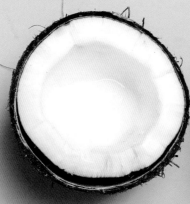
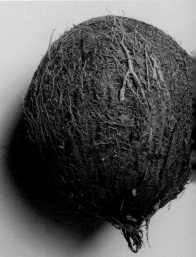

OTHER OILS, BUTTERS & FATS
TAKE YOUR PICK!

In addition to coconut oil, there are a number of other recommended options you can consider.

RED PALM OIL

When nonrefined and untreated, red palm oil is environmentally friendly (unlike hydrogenated and refined palm oil). The oil is the next-best source of MCTs after coconut oil: 40 to 50 per cent of its fatty acids are MCTs, essentially in the form of palmitic acid.

TIPS FOR USE:
• Always opt for an extra-virgin red palm oil derived from organic farming. Don't use refined oil.

OTHER OILS

The following oils are recommended due to their richness in omega-3s and their ratio of omega-3s to omega-6s:
• camelina oil
• chia seed oil
• sacha inchi oil
• rapeseed oil

TIPS FOR USE:
• Always choose first cold-pressed unrefined virgin oils.
• Store oils in the refrigerator.
• Use oils only in their raw state; the omega-3s they contain are destroyed by cooking.

COCOA BUTTER

This contains around 63 per cent saturated fats and 34 per cent omega-9s. It's one of the most stable fats due to its natural antioxidant content, and it can withstand high temperatures very well.

TIPS FOR USE:
• Choose it in block form –100 per cent pure raw cocoa butter with a certified processing method below 45°C (113°F).
• Use it grated over meals (like Parmesan), in desserts, for cooking and making chocolate (mixed with raw cacao).

GOOSE FAT AND DUCK FAT

These fats are rich in monounsaturated fatty acids that help protect the cardiovascular system. They are very good for cooking with because of their high smoke point.

TIPS FOR USE:
• Opt for high-quality organic fats without additives or preservatives.

ALSO CONSIDER ... OLIVE OIL
Olive oil supplies precious omega-9s and monounsaturated fatty acids, recognized for their cardiovascular health benefits.

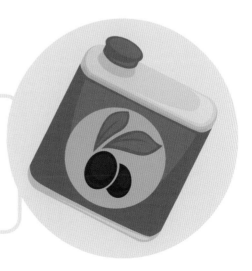

OILY NUTS & SEEDS
TO BE CONSUMED WITHOUT MODERATION (OR ALMOST!)

Rich in fats and proteins and low in carbohydrates, oily nuts play an important part in the ketogenic diet. They also supply fibre, minerals and trace elements that are essential for the healthy functioning of our bodies. Another strong point – they taste delicious and can be used in many ways and in different forms.

Just as with oils, you should opt for nuts that don't contain too many omega-6s, or, if they do, eat them sparingly. But don't deprive yourself completely of them as they have further advantages, such as being rich in certain antioxidants.

ALMONDS
The almond is a good source of fats (49 g per 100 g). More than three-quarters of its fats are monounsaturated fatty acid, in particular oleic acid, which is good for cardiovascular health. Rich in proteins (an advantage in a vegan diet), almonds also contain fibre, which is good for bowel movements and has a satiating effect. They have a remarkably high level of plant sterols, which have antioxidant and anticancer effects. Almonds are also rich in vitamins (vitamin B₂ and, most of all, the antioxidant vitamin E) and minerals, and provide an excellent source of phosphorus and magnesium. Last but not least, almonds are alkaline: they neutralize the consumption of acidifying foods such as meat.

TIPS FOR USE:
- Always choose almonds with skins and unblanched, as these are richer in fibre, vitamins and minerals.
- Opt for raw almonds that are unroasted in oil and also unsalted.
- Use as an excellent ketogenic snack.
- Crush into salads or sprinkle on fish.

GIVE THEM A SOAK!
Before consuming oily nuts and seeds, soak them in water for at least 30 minutes (or overnight). Soaking them allows the grain to 'awaken' and eliminates its antinutrients, makes it easier to digest and increases its concentration of minerals and vitamins.

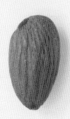
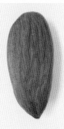
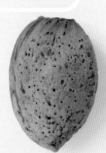
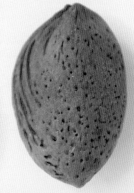

- Blend to make a 'raw' puree or a homemade plant-based milk (see page 124).
- Grind to make cakes and low-carb bread for breakfast.

MACADAMIA NUTS

Actually seeds rather than nuts, macadamias lead the way in fat richness (almost 73 g per 100 g), especially monounsaturated fatty acids (58 g). They also contain some saturated fatty acids (12g) and very few omega-6s. Macadamias are therefore ideal for daily consumption in a ketogenic diet, with a substantial level of proteins (8 g per 100 g), while being low in carbohydrates (a little less than 6 g). The nuts are also an excellent source of potassium and manganese.

TIPS FOR USE:
- Just eat them on their own or sprinkle them in salads and hot dishes.
- They are ideal for making cheese or oily caviars along with certain other superfoods.

HAZELNUTS

Hazelnuts contain less than 6 g of carbohydrates per 100 g and have a fat content of 63 g per 100 g. The nuts are especially rich in oleic acid or omega-9s (42 g) and somewhat low in omega-6s and saturated fatty acids. They are also an excellent source of antioxidants and supply many minerals, such as manganese, copper, phosphorus and magnesium, as well as vitamin E.

TIPS FOR USE:
- Eat with their brown skins on: this is where the antioxidants are concentrated.
- Eat whole as a snack or crushed into salads and soups.
- Grind, as flour or as a milk or puree.

ALSO CONSIDER ...
BRAZIL NUTS

Low in carbohydrates, brazil nuts are also very rich in selenium (a powerful antioxidant and anti-inflammatory), magnesium, phosphorus, manganese and coppe, as well as vitamins E and B_1. The nuts do, however, have a slightly less desirable level of omega-6s (23 g per 100 g), equivalent to their level of omega-9s (26 g). Don't consume too many of the nuts, no more than two to four per day, as they can contain barium, which is toxic to the liver.

TIPS FOR USE:
- Eat them whole or crushed into salads.

PECAN NUTS

With their low carbohydrate content, pecan nuts are rich in monounsaturated acids, omega-6s and saturated fatty acids. They are also a good source of antioxidants, omega-6s and minerals, including manganese, copper and zinc.

TIPS FOR USE:
- Eat them on their own or add them to porridge or salads.

SMALL OILY SEEDS

Although often overlooked in our diet, these small seeds pack an unbelievable amount of nutrients. They are low in carbohydrates and contain omega-3s, omega-6s, vitamins, fibre and minerals. Don't forget to include them in your meals!

PLEASE NOTE!
- Don't heat the seeds as this causes oxidization and makes them harmful to your health.
- Buy seeds in small quantities and store them away from light as they can oxidize quickly.
- Don't buy ground seeds. It's best to choose whole seeds and grind just the required amount yourself.

FLAXSEEDS

The main advantage of flaxseeds is their high amount of anti-inflammatory omega-3s. They are also a good source of soluble fibre – ideal for constipation as well as for slightly reducing cholesterol levels in the blood. In addition, flaxseeds supply lignans (phytoestrogens), which may help to reduce certain menopausal symptoms.

TIPS FOR USE:
- Try whole or ground.
- Sprinkle on salads.
- For constipation – drink one glass of water with a teaspoon of seeds (unground, as an exception) in the morning.

CHIA SEEDS

These seeds from Central America are low in carbohydrates and rich in fats, particularly omega-3s, in the form of alpha-linolenic acid. They also supply around 8 per cent of healthy omega-6s and are anti-inflammatory. Chia seeds contain a lot of fibre and are therefore effective against constipation and help regulate bowel movements. They are rich in proteins and antioxidants as well as in vitamins and minerals, including calcium, phosphorus, magnesium, potassium, iron, zinc and copper.

TIPS FOR USE:
- Soak the seeds in water or a plant-based milk for several hours to make a chia gel – put 1 tablespoon of freshly ground seeds in 40 ml (1½ fl oz) of water, let it stand for at least 20 minutes and then store in the fridge. It makes an excellent breakfast dish.
- Grind and mix into almond milk or coconut cream with some oily fruits and seeds to make a great breakfast dish low in carbohydrates and rich in good fats.
- To thicken porridge, soups, sauces and smoothies.
- As an oil that can be stored in the fridge.

HULLED HEMP SEEDS

The many nutritional properties of hemp seeds were only recently discovered. They are rich in high-quality proteins and fibre, easy to digest and a good source of omega-3s (around 24 per cent) and omega-6s (around 60 per cent). The seeds also supply various minerals and vitamins. And don't worry – you can't get high on hemp seeds!

TIPS FOR USE:
- Sprinkle on raw salads.
- As an oil that can be stored in the fridge.

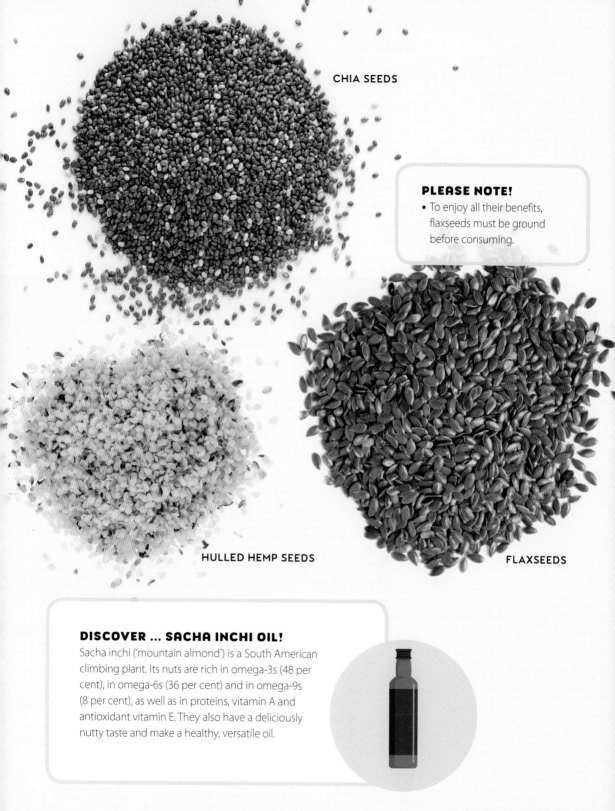

CHIA SEEDS

PLEASE NOTE!
• To enjoy all their benefits, flaxseeds must be ground before consuming.

HULLED HEMP SEEDS

FLAXSEEDS

DISCOVER ... SACHA INCHI OIL!

Sacha inchi ('mountain almond') is a South American climbing plant. Its nuts are rich in omega-3s (48 per cent), in omega-6s (36 per cent) and in omega-9s (8 per cent), as well as in proteins, vitamin A and antioxidant vitamin E. They also have a deliciously nutty taste and make a healthy, versatile oil.

EGGS
A KETOGENIC CLASSIC

Eggs are one of the key foods in the ketogenic diet: they supply fats (around 10 g per 100 g for every two eggs) and proteins (12 g per 100 g) but very few carbohydrates (less than 1 g per 100 g). In addition, the quality of the fats and proteins in eggs is very high.

The fats in eggs are mainly contained in the yolk. These are mostly monounsaturated fatty acids and known to be beneficial for cardiovascular health. The proteins in eggs are often considered by nutritionists to be the protein benchmark. In fact, they contain 22 different amino acids (including the nine essential amino acids that our bodies are not able to produce), in proportions that are perfectly balanced for the human body's requirements.

Furthermore, egg yolks are the foods highest in choline (125 mg per 100 g), an essential nutrient for the brain. Egg yolk also contains lutein, an antioxidant that appears to block or reduce the harmful effects of free radicals. And it's also a good source of vitamins (A, D, E and B, especially the prized B_{12} vitamin), trace elements and minerals (selenium, in significant quantities, phosphorus, zinc, sodium and potassium).

HOW TO CHOOSE EGGS

- Choose free-range organic eggs from hens fed on flaxseeds. These eggs contain a beneficial level of omega-3s.
- Look beyond chicken eggs! Try quails' eggs, duck eggs and goose eggs.
- Make sure eggs are fresh. They are considered to be extra fresh up to nine days after laying, and then fresh for up to 28 days. Eggs should not be consumed beyond this time period.

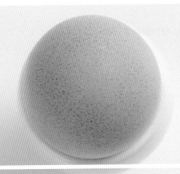

HOW TO EAT EGGS

- Omelettes, scrambled, fried, soft-boiled or poached
- Gratins, quiches, sauces, creams, crepes – but be careful not to eat too many cooked eggs. Try to use raw yolks – for example, in chocolate cream recipes.
- A couple of soft-boiled eggs for breakfast or lunch, or on an endive salad.

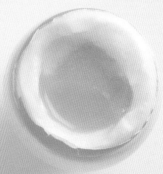

EGG SENSE!

- Two eggs provide as much protein as 100 g (3½ oz) of meat or fish.
- To enjoy the benefits of all their vitamins, minerals and very fragile omega-3s, egg yolks should be consumed soft or raw, and their whites cooked. If the yolk is overcooked, the proteins get altered and become harder to digest. It's best to eat eggs poached or soft-boiled rather than hard-boiled.

FERMENTED SOY
PAMPER YOUR INTESTINAL FLORA

Fermented soy is preferable to standard soy because fermentation increases availability of the nutrients, makes the proteins and fibre easier to digest and optimizes absorption of the micronutrients. Moreover, fermented soy provides good protective bacteria for your intestinal flora.

Soy has all the essential amino acids in the right proportions, providing an excellent alternative to animal protein. Also, soy and soy-derived products contain isoflavones (a group of phytoestrogens), in particular genistein, which may prove to be an important compound in the prevention of tumour growth. The highest levels of genistein are found in fermented foods. This is why it's important to consume only lacto-fermented soy and avoid other soy-based products, which contain too many antinutrients (see box below). You can eat lacto-fermented soy between one to three times per week but not every day.

HOW DO WE USE SOY?
- Lacto-fermented tofu is rich in proteins (on average 19 g of proteins per 100 g, almost as much as in meat). It also has very few carbohydrates (on average 1.3 g per 100 g) and around 10 g of fats. This makes it a food perfectly suited to the ketogenic diet.
- Tempeh is a cheeselike, soy-based food that comes from Indonesia. It's made by coagulating soy milk, fermented with mushrooms, and is a good source of plant proteins and fibre.

PLEASE NOTE!
The Chinese and Japanese use only fermented soy. This fermentation neutralizes the toxins and antinutrients (trypsin inhibitors) found in the beans. So, be careful to avoid soy milk and unfermented tofu blocks as well as soy flour.

- Organic natto, made from fermenting small yellow soy beans, is a popular traditional Japanese food, probably invented by Buddhist monks. Because it tastes like cheese, natto is an acquired taste! Along with tempeh, this is the healthiest soy-based food as it's the most natural and least processed (this is not a 'block' of soy). Additionally, natto is rich in vitamin K_2, which plays a key role in bone metabolism (preventing osteoporosis). However, as it's richer in carbohydrates than lacto-fermented tofu, natto must be consumed in reasonable quantities in a ketogenic diet and is better suited to a low-carb diet.

ALSO CONSIDER ...
UNPASTEURIZED RICE MISO
A very healthy food to use as a condiment in small quantities, rice miso is rich in electrolytes. It lends itself to a ketogenic diet, where hydration is paramount. This miso is also great for restoring the balance of the intestinal flora.

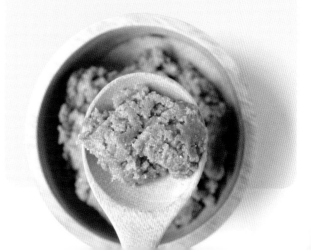

MEAT
TO BE CONSUMED – IN MODERATION!

Due to its fat and protein content and lack of carbohydrates, as a general rule meat has a special place in the ketogenic diet. Remember, though, that meat is pro-inflammatory, and so you should not eat too much of it.

Although less rich in fats than red meat, white meat (veal, rabbit) and poultry (chicken, turkey, guinea fowl, duck, ostrich) are also less rich in iron and pro-oxidant compounds than red meat.

PLEASE NOTE!
Plant proteins, eggs and small fish are better options for your health.

HOW TO CHOOSE MEAT
Always choose good-quality meat. Opt for organic meat derived from free-range, grass-fed animals (they will be richer in good fats and so contain omega-3s).

Avoid supermarket meat, if possible, as the animals are fed mainly on feed meal high in omega-6s, which means the meat has a significant proportion of arachidonic acid – and no omega-3s!

THE RIGHT WAY TO EAT MEAT
- Always consume meat in moderation. It's better to eat it once a week, or even once a month, or even avoid it completely to become healthier!
- Have meat for lunch rather than in the evening.
- Be careful with your cooking methods. Avoid cooking at very high temperatures and especially grilling (including barbecues), which create carcinogenic compounds. The proteins in the meat are denatured when the cooking temperature exceeds 100°C (212°F), and cooking at such high temperatures creates pro-oxidant and carcinogenic molecules. It's preferable to cook the meat at lower temperatures, for example in a steam cooker, or stew the meat gently for a long time.
- Always serve your meat with a large portion of fibre-rich green vegetables (such as salad, leeks, endives, cabbage or courgettes), to compensate for the meat's acidifying effect.

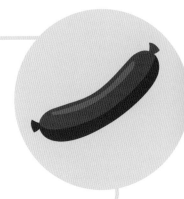

ALSO CONSIDER ... LACTO-FERMENTED MEAT!
This meat and its fat are simply preserved using only salt. Go for real, organic-quality dry sausages, for example, made only with fat, meat and salt. Lacto-fermented dry sausages made with pork or duck are a good option and may contain some omega-3s if the animals were free-range, not fed on feed meal (with corn and soy), but rather fed on a vegetarian diet and possibly flaxseeds. Also consider raw ham, such as high-quality Parma ham.

FISH
YES, BUT NOT JUST ANY KIND

Small oily fish can play an important role in the ketogenic diet as they have no carbohydrates, are more or less rich in fats (omega-3s) and are a good source of proteins. They also supply minerals, trace elements and vitamins.

HOW TO CHOOSE FISH
• Opt for anchovies that are free from pollutants, such as polychlorinated biphenyl (PCB), pesticides, mercury, lead and cadmium found in fish and sea food. As for larger fish, try to exclude tuna, salmon and other large predator fish of this type.
• Also consider fish preserved in olive oil and in glass jars: ideally anchovies and, from time to time, sardines or mackerel.
• Raw sardine fillets 'cooked' in lemon and olive oil are also good as this preserves their heat-sensitive omega-3s.

PLEASE NOTE!
Not all oily fish are the same. The largest (such as swordfish, shark, tuna and salmon) feed on smaller fish, and so are full of pollutants and heavy metals, especially mercury, a powerful neurotoxin. To avoid this problem, eat only small oily fish, such as anchovies (ideally), sardines and mackerel.

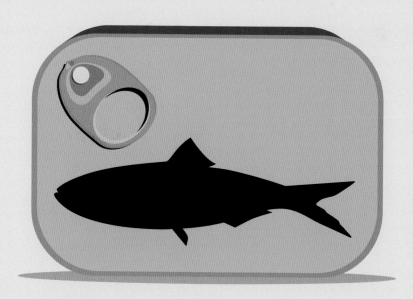

SEAWEED
AN EXCEPTIONALLY RICH RESOURCE

Extremely rich in what are called 'complete' proteins (23 per cent of its weight), seaweed contains all the essential amino acids.

Seaweed also contains ten to twenty times more minerals than land vegetables. In particular, seaweed offers large concentrations of calcium, magnesium, phosphorus, manganese and iron.

This abundance of mineral salts puts seaweed at the top of the list of remineralizing foods. An alkaline food par excellence, it helps to neutralize the body's acidification, linked to excessive consumption of animal proteins and grains. It also contains chlorophyll (good for acid-base balance and detoxification of the blood), vitamins (B9, C and A), active substances for toxin elimination and antioxidant substances such as phlorotannins or polyphenols, and a high iodine content (very important for healthy thyroid function).

Seaweed also supplies high-quality polyunsaturated fatty acids – omega-3s in the form of eicosapentaenoic acid (EPA), docosahexaenoic acid (DHA) and gamma-linolenic acid (GLA), depending on the type of seaweed). These are very similar to the omega-3s found in oily fish. Last but not least, seaweed is rich in fibre. This abundance is helpful for bowel movements and provides a feeling of fullness. So, there are plenty of good reasons to include seaweed in your daily diet!

HOW TO CHOOSE SEAWEED?

- Fresh seaweed is best. If this isn't possible, you can get it in the form of seaweed flakes in organic stores. These are guaranteed in terms of toxicological and microbiological criteria, subject to strict controls and grown in protected areas.
- You could try sea lettuce, nori, wakame, kombu, dulse or salicornia (plants, such as samphire, that grow partly immersed in water and are not, strictly speaking, seaweed).

HOW TO USE SEAWEED

- As a seaweed tartare (found in organic stores – or make it yourself, see page 119).
- In stocks and soups.
- Seaweed flakes in salads.

ENERGY BOOSTER!

By consuming a small quantity of seaweed every day or several times a week, you'll soon notice an increase in your energy, which may indicate that you were deficient in iodine and perhaps other minerals too.

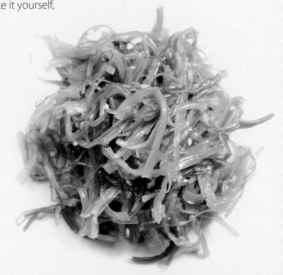

VEGETABLES
LET'S SORT THESE OUT!

As an indispensable source of fibre, vitamins, minerals and phytonutrients, vegetables play a major role in the ketogenic diet. But be careful - not just any kind!

The carbohydrate content of vegetables can vary widely, with some having less that 2 g of carbohydrates per 100 g (cooked spinach) and others nearly 17 g (sweet potatoes).

PLEASE NOTE!
The vegetables highest in carbohydrates are root vegetables (which have grown underground), such as sweet potato, potato and parsnip. They should be avoided.

CAULIFLOWER
The cauliflower is a favourite ketogenic food. In addition to its low carbohydrate content, it makes for an ideal alternative to many starches.

TIPS FOR USE:
• Puree it to replace potatoes.
• When grated and cooked, use it just like rice.
• When grated and raw, cauliflower has a similar texture to semolina, and is ideal for low-carb tabbouleh recipes.

COURGETTES
The courgette is another favourite vegetable of the ketogenic diet. It's 95 per cent water, low in carbohydrates and rich in potassium and rutin, a phenolic compound from the flavonoid group that promotes healthy blood pressure and is also an antioxidant.

TIPS FOR USE:
• Cut into thin strips – courgettes make a great substitute for spaghetti.
• Grated raw in salad.

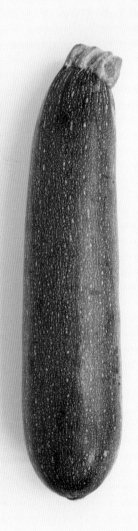
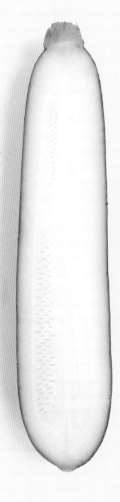

OTHER LOW-CARB VEGETABLES

- Green leafy vegetables: lettuce, endives, chard, watercress, lamb's lettuce, purslane, baby spinach, curly endive, rocket
- Cruciferous vegetables: green cabbage, broccoli, kale, brussels sprouts, romanesco, red cabbage
- Additonal vegetables: cucumber, tomato, radish, black radish, raw celery sticks, leeks, celeriac, green and red peppers, artichoke, asparagus, fennel
- Mushrooms (except shiitake, which contains 7 g of carbohydrates per 100 g) to be eaten in small quantities
- Sprouted mung beans (in salads) and all sprouted seeds, including alfalfa, cress, leek and radish

THE RIGHT WAY TO EAT VEGETABLES

Always opt for vegetables in season, local (if possible) and organically grown in order to avoid pesticides, which unfortunately are not concentrated only in the skins. This way, your vegetables will be much more nutritious. Always choose quality over quantity!

- You could also use organic frozen vegetables (uncooked). However, be careful with tinned vegetables as they can contain added sugars.
- Also think about vegetables preserved in oil (such as artichokes and sun-dried tomatoes) but always check the list of ingredients on the label.

ALSO CONSIDER ... LACTO-FERMENTED VEGETABLES

Food when fermented is transformed by microorganisms, which synthesize their enzymes. They are catalysts in this biochemical process, allowing the release of energy and the rejection of many different substances – both actions that are useful for our bodies. The process takes place anaerobically (without oxygen), with the exception of microorganisms at work in all lacto-fermented vegetables.

By regularly eating small quantities of raw lacto-fermented vegetables (in salads), you naturally take in probiotics (lactic bacteria), thereby taking care of your microbiota for the proper functioning of your immune system.

Another advantage: A lacto-fermented vegetable contains ten times more vitamin C than the same vegetable freshly picked. The transformation by the bacteria also makes the food easier to digest. Additionally, lacto-fermentation converts a part of the carbohydrates into lactic acid, thereby reducing the carbohydrate content.

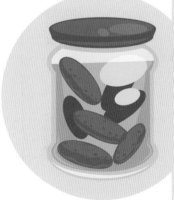

HOW TO USE THEM

- Ready-to-use in jars, preserved in salt, in the fresh produce section in organic stores: cabbage (sauerkraut), celery, turnip, leek, cucumber, carrot or beetroot. The lacto-fermented vegetables in glass jars that are not in the fresh produce section are pasteurized, and of no interest as they have very low levels of probiotics.
- Make them yourself at home.

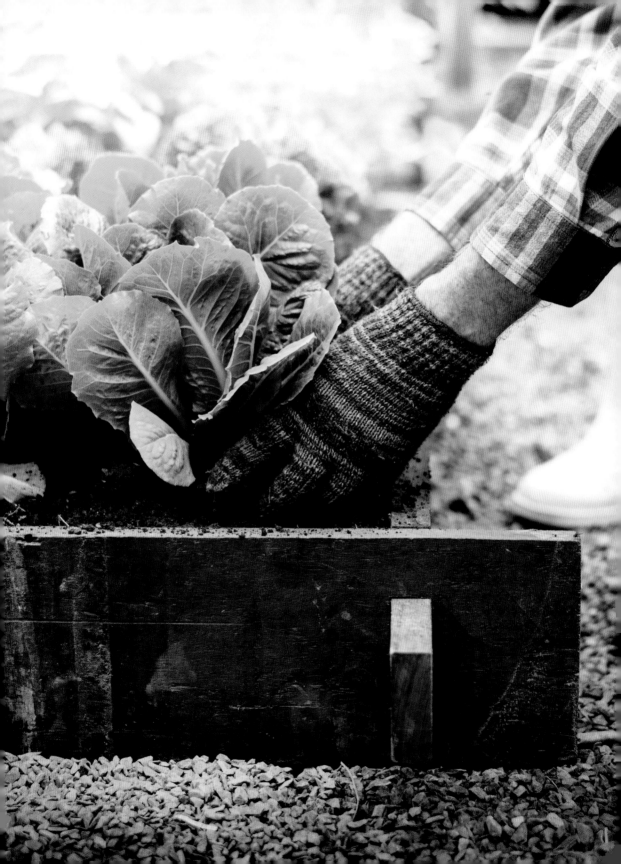

FRUIT
A LIMITED LIST

Fruit by definition is sweet and therefore rich in carbohydrates. And so, in the ketogenic diet, eating fruit is avoided as much as possible. There are some notable exceptions, however.

AVOCADO
Contrary to common belief, the avocado is actually a fruit, even if it's often used as a vegetable. In addition to its low level of carbohydrates (3 g per 100 g) and its 5–6 g of fibre, the avocado is an excellent source of fat (16 g per 100 g). It also contains many minerals essential to the ketogenic diet, with potassium at the top of the list. Avocados also have a high content of certain vitamins (in particular B_9 and E), as well as vitamin-like nutrients such as choline.

The avocado is a high-alkaline food and therefore ideal for regulating your acid-base balance. The fatty acid composition is comparable to that of olive oil, due to its richness in oleic acid, and the average content of monounsaturated fatty acids (omega-9s) in avocados is 76 per cent. The fruit also contains many antioxidants, including phytosterols (beta-sitosterol, campesterol and stigmasterol), vitamin E (tocopherols and tocotrienols), tannins and pigments (chlorophyll, polyphenols, proanthocyanidins and carotenoids), squalene and stanols.

HOW TO USE AVOCADOS
- Crushed into guacamole, with homemade seaweed tartare.
- Sliced into salads, with soft-boiled eggs.
- With meat.
- Sweetened with berries.
- As a chocolate mousse – it's tasty and impressive (see page 122).

CHOOSING AVOCADOS
Opt for organic Haas avocados, and buy when in season (from southern Europe).

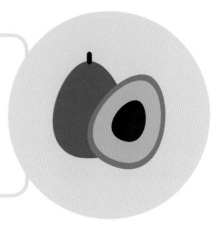

COCONUT

This fruit – actually an enormous seed – is not only very low in carbohydrates (less than 4 g per 100 g in fresh coconuts and around 9 g in dried coconuts) but also an excellent source of fats (more than 35 g per 100 g in fresh coconuts and more than 56 g in dried coconuts). Coconut oil is composed of saturated fatty acids, in particular medium-chain fatty acids (lauric acid).

The coconut also contains fibre and healthy minerals, such as potassium, iron, manganese and selenium, and is a good source of selenium. As a flour (fresh coconut, dried and ground into a very fine powder), its carbohydrate content is 20 g per 100 g, which is low for a flour. It has no gluten and can be used in small quantities as its richness in fibre (around 45 g per 100 g) means it greatly expands. Although helpful in cases of constipation, the coconut isn't necessarily appreciated by all intestines! If yours are irritable, you will need to reduce the quantities.

Coconut milk and coconut cream are excellent alternatives to milk and cream. They are low in carbohydrates but high in good fats.

PLEASE NOTE!

Coconut cream is richer in fats than coconut milk, which contains more (coconut) water.

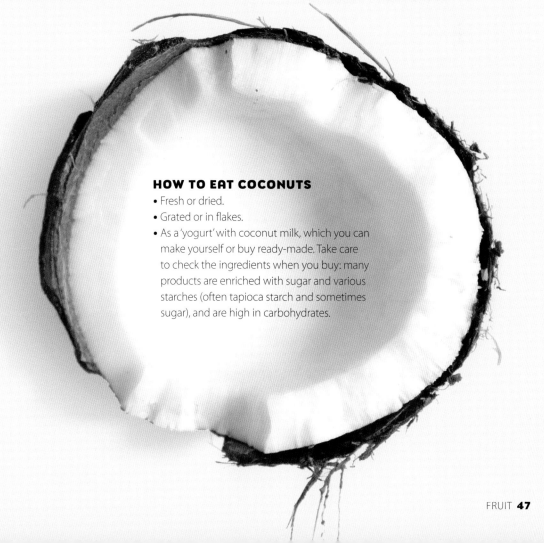

HOW TO EAT COCONUTS

- Fresh or dried.
- Grated or in flakes.
- As a 'yogurt' with coconut milk, which you can make yourself or buy ready-made. Take care to check the ingredients when you buy: many products are enriched with sugar and various starches (often tapioca starch and sometimes sugar), and are high in carbohydrates.

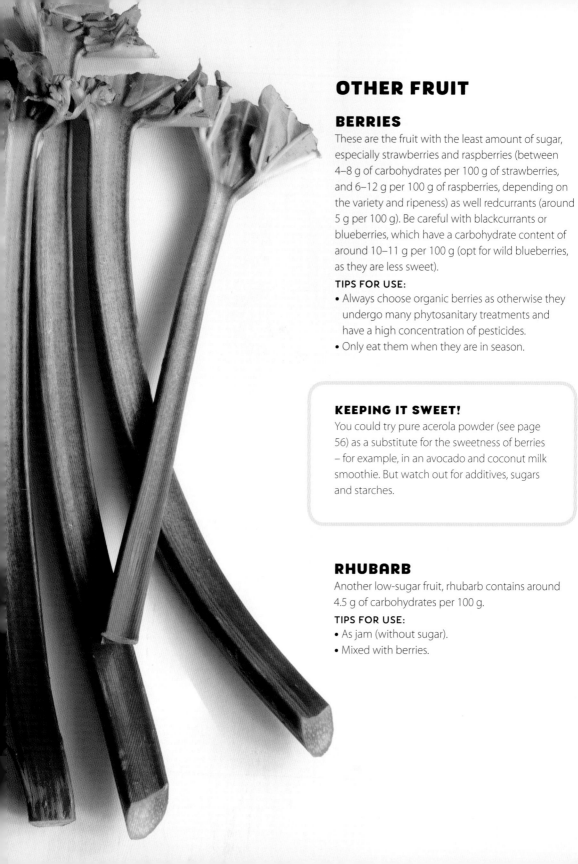

OTHER FRUIT

BERRIES

These are the fruit with the least amount of sugar, especially strawberries and raspberries (between 4–8 g of carbohydrates per 100 g of strawberries, and 6–12 g per 100 g of raspberries, depending on the variety and ripeness) as well redcurrants (around 5 g per 100 g). Be careful with blackcurrants or blueberries, which have a carbohydrate content of around 10–11 g per 100 g (opt for wild blueberries, as they are less sweet).

TIPS FOR USE:

- Always choose organic berries as otherwise they undergo many phytosanitary treatments and have a high concentration of pesticides.
- Only eat them when they are in season.

KEEPING IT SWEET!

You could try pure acerola powder (see page 56) as a substitute for the sweetness of berries – for example, in an avocado and coconut milk smoothie. But watch out for additives, sugars and starches.

RHUBARB

Another low-sugar fruit, rhubarb contains around 4.5 g of carbohydrates per 100 g.

TIPS FOR USE:

- As jam (without sugar).
- Mixed with berries.

BLACK AND RED OLIVES

Low in carbohydrates (less than 2 g per 100 g), black and red olives are rich in fats (around 14 g per 100 g), particularly oleic acid (omega-9s). They contain natural polyphenols, which provide many health benefits, and antioxidants, especially carotenes and phenolic compounds. Olives also contain a significant level of vitamin E.

HOW TO CHOOSE OLIVES

- Preferably choose black olives from Nyons or organic Greek Kalamata 'red' olives preserved in salt and unpasteurized – as these will have been preserved with lacto-fermentation (lactic acid), which has many benefits for our intestinal flora.
- Read labels carefully or, if in doubt, contact the producer directly.
- Avoid green olives, which are olives picked when still unripe, just as they are acidifying.

HOW TO EAT OLIVES

- As an appetizer with drinks.
- In salads.
- As tapenade.
- In an omelette.

PLEASE NOTE!

Some people have an intolerance for olives: it isn't because a food is generally considered healthy that it's also good for you specifically. You should also listen to your body's reactions.

LEMON

Lemons are recommended because of their antioxidant effect (in particular due to the d-limonene content in lemon zest) and their high content of vitamin C. They contain pectin, coumarin (essential oils), bioflavonoids and carotenoids (antioxidants). Thanks to its many enzymes, lemon juice detoxifies the liver and, by stimulating the liver, it helps to eliminate toxins. However, the juice is acidifying and attacks tooth enamel, which can lead to demineralization in the long term.

TIPS FOR USE:

- To detox: on an empty stomach, drink a glass of warm water with a few drops of lemon (not for longer than three weeks and avoid in winter).
- As a replacement for vinegar.

PLEASE NOTE!

Although the lemon is recognized as being alkalizing, not everyone can metabolize its acids. You need a strong enzymatic capacity to be able to manage lemon acids, so it's always better to consume lemons or lemon juice only in the spring and summer, and never in excess.

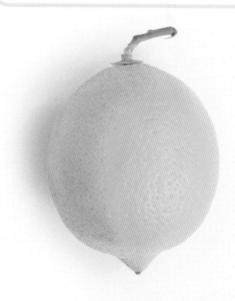

SEASONINGS

SPICES

HEALTHY SPRINKLES

Spices have a lot of healthy qualities. They contain many active substances (phytonutrients, essential oils, antioxidants), which fight aging and protect our immune system with proven anticancer effects.

Every spice and medicinal herb contains one or more active substances that act on our bodies. Broadly speaking, they ease digestion, cleanse our digestive system and help to increase our intake of antioxidants. Some also have anti-inflammatory properties. This is true, for example, of turmeric, ginger, cumin and nutmeg. Almost all herbs and spices have the advantage of being low in carbohydrates, so they can be included in a ketogenic diet without restrictions. The exceptions are ginger, garlic and onion, although, if eaten in small quantities, they don't present a problem. In fact, these are powerful antioxidants and it would be a shame to deprive ourselves of them.

THE RIGHT WAY TO EAT SPICES

- Add a pinch of spices to every dish and enjoy all their health benefits.
- They are delicious with coconut oil or coconut cream (try them with chicken, lacto-fermented tofu or cauliflower).
- Mix together ground turmeric, cardamom, cumin, ginger, coriander and coconut milk – delicious on cauliflower tabbouleh, on cabbage and on other vegetables.
- Blend fresh turmeric with coconut oil. This lightly spiced orange coconut butter tastes great and has strong protective properties for our cells.

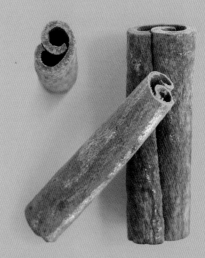

REPLACE SUGAR WITH ... CINNAMON

Cinnamon is particularly beneficial as it's rich in antioxidants and has a glucose-lowering effect. Enjoy its benefits by adding it to fruit and to replace sugar. A cinnamon tea with a few raw cocoa beans or a piece of 100 per cent raw cacao makes a delicious snack and can be enjoyed after meals.

AROMATIC HERBS
A LITTLE EXTRA FLAVOUR

Like spices, fresh or dry herbs help to enhance the flavour of your dishes. They also provide healthy antioxidants, some of which aid digestion. Generally speaking, their carbohydrate content is negligible.

THE RIGHT WAY TO EAT AROMATIC HERBS

• In summer, as well as in winter, bring a little touch of green and extra flavour to all your dishes with a few herbs, such as parsley, coriander, mint, basil, tarragon, nettles, thyme, rosemary and bay leaf.
• Fresh is better, but you can also opt for frozen or dried herbs

UNPASTEURIZED RICE MISO

This is a very healthy food made from fermented miso and rich in probiotics that you can include in your daily diet in small quantities.

TIPS FOR USE:
• To prepare the famous miso soup.
• To season sautéed vegetables, make a salad dressing or flavour soups.

PLEASE NOTE!

Be careful not to boil rice miso or it could lose its healthy properties. Preferably choose the unpasteurized kind: it will be rich in vitamins, enzymes, electrolytes and good bacteria.

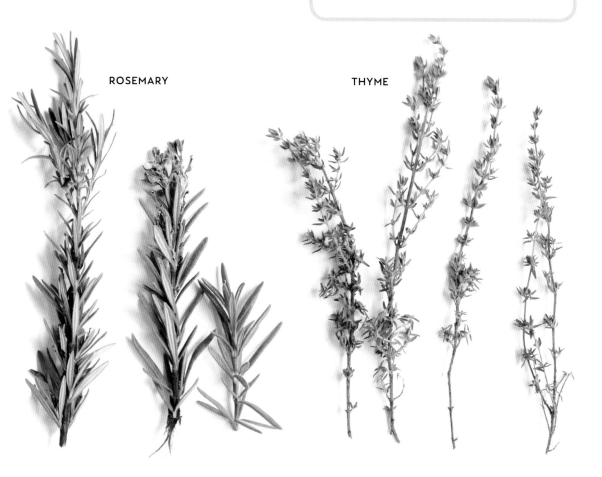

ROSEMARY

THYME

VINEGARS
THE TOP THREE

Made by fermenting alcoholic liquids or fruit, vinegars have the great benefit of lowering blood sugar, which is perfect for a ketogenic diet. However, not all vinegars are the same, so here are the ones that are recommended.

COCONUT VINEGAR

This is made using a double fermentation process of the sap or water of the coconut. The first fermentation, with the help of bacteria present in the air, makes coconut wine. This is then fermented a second time with a 'mother' of vinegar composed of acetic acid bacteria, which transforms the alcohol into acetic acid. The result is a vinegar rich in probiotics from fermentation but also rich in minerals (especially potassium) from the coconut and amino acids. The vinegar contains no sugar. It's not always easy to find but usually available online or in organic stores.

UME PLUM VINEGAR

Also known as umeboshi vinegar, this is made from a variety of plum, popular in Japan, that is dried and lacto-fermented with shiso leaves. Because of the way it's made, the vinegar is rich in probiotics that are healthy for the microbiota. You can find the vinegar in organic stores or online. It's an excellent, slightly sweet vinegar with a carbohydrate level of 4–5 g per 100 ml.

CIDER VINEGAR

For use in the ketogenic diet, cider vinegar must be organic, unpasteurized and sulphite-free. Its acetic fermentation process with bacteria produces high levels of potassium and antiseptic qualities. Cider vinegar is also less acidic than wine vinegar.

PLEASE NOTE!

Don't forget that vinegar is an acidifying food. If you have hyperchlorhydria (high stomach acid), it's best not to have too much vinegar and to opt for the lacto-fermented kind.

Anyone suffering from gastritis, gastro-oesophageal reflux (acid reflux) or ulcers should avoid vinegar.

KEY SUPERFOODS

These are plants with a high nutritional density - in other words very rich in phytonutrients, antioxidants, vitamins and minerals, and with remarkable health properties. These foods are able to supplement nutritional deficiencies and should be consumed in small quantities. Here are a few examples that you can easily include in a ketogenic diet.

CACAO

Cacao can be part of a low-carbohydrate diet, as long as it's 'raw'. This kind of cacao has not been heated above 45°C (113°F), which preserves all its original nutritional richness. Raw cacao is one of the foods richest in nutrients, including vitamins B2 and B3 and minerals. In particular, it has five to six times more magnesium than cooked cacao, as well as significant amounts of phosphorus, iron, copper and potassium. It's also a good source of zinc, an important nutrient for the immune system.

This little bean is also very rich in antioxidants. It contains polyphenols as well as flavonoids, which make up to 10 per cent of its total composition. Cacao is also an excellent source of the mood-boosting compound theobromine and contains neurotransmitters, such as serotonin and phenethylamine (PEA), which play a role in controlling psychological stability. Raw cacao helps to combat bad cholesterol, reduces blood pressure and thins the blood, as well as improving insulin sensitivity.

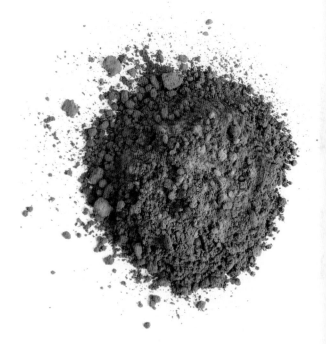

HOW TO CHOOSE CACAO

- Look for organic raw cacao (powder, bars or beans).
- Only consume 100 per cent raw cacao bars, available in organic stores. Avoid standard chocolate bars as they will always have sugar, even with 70 per cent cacao content.

THE RIGHT WAY TO EAT CACAO

- One or two squares make a very healthy snack, to be enjoyed every day, along with green tea, cinnamon herbal tea or maté.
- For those who find this cacao too bitter, sweeten it by drizzling on a little kitul syrup. This is an ideal way to get used to the rather unusual taste, before giving up sugar completely.

BLOND PSYLLIUM
AN ALLY FOR HEALTHY BOWEL MOVEMENTS

With a fibre content of 80 g per 100 g, blond psyllium (or 'Indian plantain') is particularly recommended for fighting constipation. In fact, constipation may be an unwanted side-effect when transitioning to a ketogenic diet, especially if you don't include enough oily fruit and seeds with their skins and fibre-rich vegetables while continuing to eat meat. Blond psyllium regulates bowel movements so is also helpful in tackling diarrhoea, and it plays a very useful role in lowering the glycemic index (GI). The plant doesn't contain any fats and has a relatively low level of proteins (8 g per 100 g).

PLEASE NOTE!

Always drink lots of water after absorbing psyllium to avoid obstructing the digestive tract. Increase the dose of psyllium gradually, from 1 teaspoon to 2 tablespoons per day to be taken in two doses.

HOW TO CHOOSE BLOND PSYLLIUM

- It can easily be found in the food supplement section in organic stores.
- In powder form, it can be diluted into a liquid for its effect on the digestive system. The mixture forms a protective and regulating gel in the stomach.

HOW TO CONSUME BLOND PSYLLIUM

- As a thickener for low-carbohydrate breads, crepes or cakes.
- As a cream with coconut milk and spices – delicious as a dessert.
- To bind or thicken hot sauces.

PLANT PROTEIN POWDER

Protein powders don't have the acidifying effect of meat. They contain all the essential amino acids, are very rich in enzymes and easy to digest. They are highly nutritious, hypotoxic (dairy free, gluten free and free of whey and colouring) and easily assimilated (depending on the brand, the assimilation level can be as high as 98 per cent).

THEY CAN BE HELPFUL IN REACHING PROTEIN INTAKE TARGETS FOR:

- Vegans and vegetarians and people wanting to reduce their consumption of meat without the risk of deficiencies.
- People who have difficulty in digesting animal protein due to inflammatory diseases, especially of the digestive tract.
- Athletes who need high-quality proteins for muscle recovery.
- Older people who have a low appetite or suffer from sarcopenia (loss of muscle mass, which can begin as early as around the age of 45).
- Adolescents, as a breakfast supplement to promote growth.

HOW TO CHOOSE PLANT PROTEINS

- Choose organic plant proteins that are raw, pure, 100 per cent natural and bio-sprouted without gluten. Check their assimilation levels, which can vary between 50 and 98 per cent, depending on the protein or proteins used.

PLEASE NOTE!

Make sure you don't exceed the daily dose as excess proteins take you out of ketosis. This happens because the body then uses proteins to make glucose via the mechanism of gluconeogenesis.

- Read the labels carefully and preferably choose plain, pure plant proteins or with only cacao, vanilla or a little stevia added for sweetness. Several internet sites are beginning to offer these.

HOW TO CONSUME PLANT PROTEINS
In powder form in your porridge at breakfast (2 tablespoons are the equivalent of two eggs).

SPROUTED LEGUMES & SEEDS
Sprouted legumes allow you to make the most of their benefits. In fact, thanks to the process of germination, the carbohydrate level of legumes (on average 17 g per 100 g) decreases when sprouted. Their GI also lowers, which means they can be included in small portions in a ketogenic diet. In addition, the germination process makes them more digestible by eliminating antinutrients. They also have a high satiety effect and are full of vitamins, especially from the B group. In sprouted form, lentils or chickpeas are also an excellent source of essential amino acids, vitamins and minerals, and most of all they are fabulously rich in enzymes.

But don't limit yourself to sprouted legumes! All seeds, such as alfalfa, leeks, cress and radish, can be included in a ketogenic diet. They are all rich in chlorophyll, enzymes, minerals, vitamins and essential amino acids. If you consumer seeds in their simple form, proteins, trace elements and vitamins are fully assimilated and in record time. Proteins are converted to free amino acids, which are directly assimilated. The vitamin content multiplies by ten (even by a thousand for some), especially with vitamins C, A, E and group B. New nutrients appear, including carotenoids. Seeds are not only highly alkalizing, they are also more alive and filled with bio-photons (small light emissions produced and used by all living organisms).

TIPS FOR USE:
- Raw in salads
- As a garnish on hot dishes

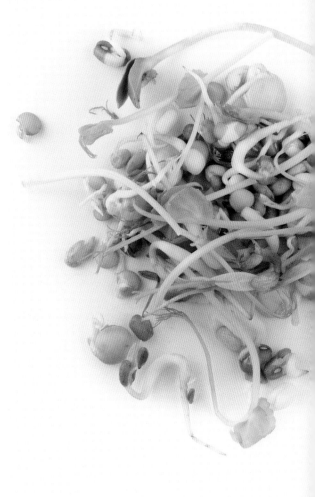

OTHER SUPERFOODS

ACAI

This small South American berry comes from a species of palm tree from the Aracaceae family. It's especially rich in antioxidants (polyphenols) and fatty acids (32 per cent) – mainly oleic acid (a monounsaturated fat) as well as linoleic acid (polyunsaturated) and palmitic acid (saturated fat). Furthermore, acai berries are a good source of vitamin E and dietary fibre. They also contain vitamins A, B_1, B_2, B_3 and C and are a significant source of iron and magnesium. This is a superfood all athletes should include in their diets.

TIPS FOR USE:
• Consume it in powder form, which can be stored for around three weeks in the fridge.
• In a soup, in oily purees or chia puddings, where 1 teaspoon is sufficient. Acai is violet in colour and will make your dishes look great, too!

PURE ACEROLA

Acerola is a small cherry that is extremely rich in vitamin C, a vitamin that acts on the immune system's resistance to attacks, on fatigue and on improving collagen quality required for our skin and intestinal lining.

TIPS FOR USE:
• Always choose pure acerola powder, containing no excipients.
• On a daily basis, take 1 teaspoon of acerola diluted in a glass of water – and also use as a snack drink.

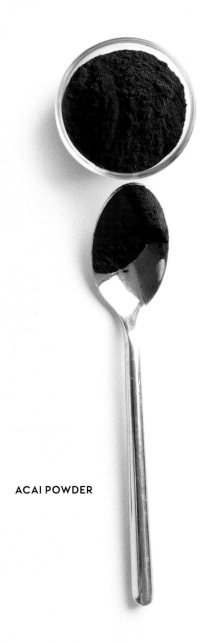

ACAI POWDER

> **PLEASE NOTE!**
> Don't exceed 1 teaspoon per day, as acerola is high in carbohydrates. It will supplement any gaps in your vitamin C intake, which is important in a ketogenic diet as you will be eating very little fruit.

CAMU CAMU

This little fruit, native to Peru, is particularly rich in vitamin C as well as in antioxidants. And it's lower in carbohydrates than acerola.

TIPS FOR USE:
- Add 1 teaspoon to a glass of water or mix it into an almond puree.

SPIRULINA

This microalga is known for its significant content of high-quality plant proteins, for its high levels of easily assimilated iron and for its many vitamins, especially from the B group, as well as vitamin K, beta-carotene and vitamin E. Spirulina also contains chlorophyll (the green blood in plants, with detoxifying properties) and phycocyanin, a blue pigment specific to cyanobacteria. Phycocyanin content is an important element to look for when choosing spirulina. This pigment is increasingly becoming a focus of medical research: it's primarily an important stimulant for the immune system. It also has antioxidant, anti-inflammatory and liver-protecting effects, and induces haematopoiesis, which is the formation and renewal of blood cells.

On average, by dry weight, spirulina contains up to 70 per cent proteins, 15–25 per cent carbohydrates and up to 11 per cent fats.

TIPS FOR USE:
- Always choose high-quality, artisanal spirulinam which has undergone a low-temperature drying process and been grown in ponds, tested to ensure no toxicity. In fact, as spirulina absorbs all metals from its growing environment, you could be at risk from toxicity if you consume low-quality uncertified spirulina.
- Try 1 teaspoon of spirulina flakes in half an avocado – it's energizing and delicious!

NUTSEDGE

A tuber found in the Mediterranean, nutsedge is also known as 'tiger nut' or 'earth almond'. Naturally gluten free, it adds a gently sweet taste to your recipes, without the need to add sugar. It has a high carbohydrate content (around 49–63 g per 100 g), but, like coconut flour, its richness in fibre (16–33 g of fibre per 100 g) keeps its insulin index low (35 on the GI). Nutsedge is good for bowel movements as well as being an excellent source of minerals (potassium, magnesium, phosphorus and iron) and fatty acids (25 per cent, and mainly omega-9s). Its protein content is around 5 g.

TIPS FOR USE:
- One or two nuts are enough to satisfy a small sugar craving. Check to make sure there's no added sugar in the packet.
- As a flour in cakes, low-carb biscuits or in your breakfast porridge. However, don't eat more than 1 tablespoon of nutsedge flour per day as it has a high carbohydrate content.

NUTSEDGE

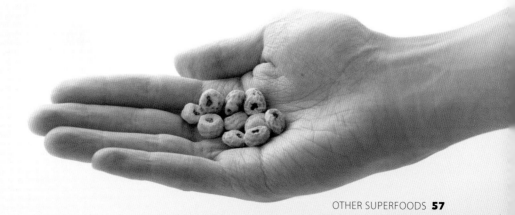

SUGAR & SUGAR PRODUCTS
SOME IDEAL SUBSTITUTES FOR YOUR TRANSITION TOWARDS A KETOGENIC DIET

The ketogenic diet tries to cut out sugar in all its forms. But it's hard to completely give up the sugary taste you have been used to since childhood! Help is at hand, though, with these sugar alternatives.

True addiction to sugar does actually exist and the less sugar you eat, the less you'll crave it. Fortunately, there are some low glycemic index (GI) sugar substitutes to help you as you transition towards a ketogenic diet. They make a good alternative to refined sugar, which has had all its minerals removed, is addictive and promotes weight gain, which can lead to type 2 diabetes and obesity. The following are some possible options to help you during your transitional phase.

COCONUT SUGAR

An artisanal product made from the sap of coconut palm flowers, coconut sugar is produced in the traditional way in Indonesia and the Philippines. It has a low GI of 35 (compared to glucose at 100 and sucrose at 70), but the main difference is that this is a living sugar with lots of minerals, such as zinc, potassium, phosphorus, copper, magnesium and iron, as well as vitamins B_1 and C.

TIPS FOR USE:
- In pastries.
- In porridge.
- To sweeten hot drinks.

KITUL SAP

This is extracted from a tropical tree called *Caryota urens* or sugar palm, which grows in the humid coastal regions of Sri Lanka and south India. Kitul sap has a low GI (45) and is also a living sugar, containing lots of minerals (including zinc, potassium, calcium, magnesium and iron) and vitamins (B_1, C and B_{12}). It also has a delicious taste of caramel.

TIPS FOR USE:
- One drizzle is enough to flavour a dessert.
- Once opened, store the bottle in the fridge.

ALSO DISCOVER ... COCONUT SYRUP
This syrup has a smooth texture and a low GI (45) and is very sweet.

YACON

Known also as 'pear of the earth', the yacon is a tuberous plant native to the Andean countries Peru, Bolivia and Ecuador, which likes high altitude – up to 2,000 m (6,562 ft). It's distinguished by its richness in fructo-oligosaccharides (FOS), which are sugars that the human metabolism cannot break down, and so are not assimilated. However, they are excellent prebiotics, promoting the intestinal flora's good bacteria, which are essential for appetite and weight management. The yacon tuber is squeezed to extract an intensely sweet syrup (25 g of yacon can replace 150 g of sugar), containing only 1–4 g of carbohydrates per portion of 100 g of fresh root (according to the International Potato Center in Peru). Yacon is also rich in potassium, providing 185–296 mg per 100 g. With a GI as low as 1, it could be used as an alternative to stevia (see below).

TIPS FOR USE:

• In powder or syrup form, yacon is perfectly suitable as a sweetener in a low-carb diet.

ALSO DISCOVER …
YACON LEAVES

Yacon leaves are excellent as herbal teas. They don't have a sweet taste and their GI is zero. They promote the regulation of sugar levels in our bodies as well as weight loss. In Japan, the 'tea of the Andes' is marketed by a Japanese yacon association, which recommends regular consumption of this tea to diabetic patients.

ORGANIC NATURAL STEVIA

Stevia comes from a plant native to Latin America. It has zero calories and therefore zero carbohydrates. In stevia's natural state, its green leaves, with hints of anise or liquorice, have a sweetening power fifteen to twenty times greater than that of white sugar.

TIPS FOR USE:

• In leaves or powder form from organic stores. Choose natural stevia made from the entire

PLEASE NOTE!

Since 2009, stevia has also been marketed in the form of a white substance with a sweetening power 300 times greater than white sugar. It's obtained by isolating stevia's sweetening molecules from its other compounds – a refining process that totally destroys the plant's natural balance. The resulting white powder is factory-made from intensively farmed raw materials, 80 per cent of which comes from China, and is nothing like the healthy food that this plant really is. Avoid this if you care about your health!

plant, organic, green in colour and pure. It should not be an extract of stevia even if it's organic, or an ingredient combined with other synthetic sweeteners, which is often the case with products found in supermarkets.

• Make the syrup yourself from the entire plant. Cover the whole or crushed stevia leaves with fresh water for a few days. Filter this macerate to get a very sweet liquid with a less pronounced liquorice–anise taste. You can store this macerate in the fridge to use for your desserts. A drizzle is more than enough.

EVEN HEALTHIER
'SWEETENING' TIPS

• For 'sweetening', think also of using spices such as cinnamon or vanilla to sweeten your dishes.
• You could also try ready-to-use lemon or orange skins or zest, which can be found in organic stores (in the spice section). Or, even better, simply use fresh lemon zest.
• Some 'flours', such as almond powder, hazelnut powder, coconut flour or even nutsedge flour, can also provide a pleasant and natural sweet taste.
• Think also of certain superfoods with a slightly sweet flavour, such as maca, raw carob (which can replace cacao) or even lucuma (which tastes like dried dates). Use these only in small quantities as they have a higher carbohydrate content.

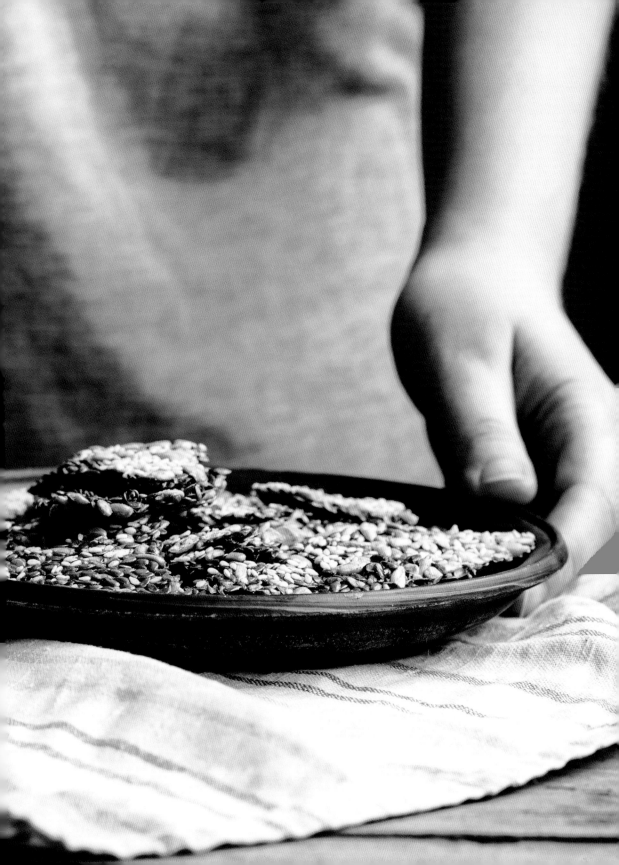

FORBIDDEN FOODS

The ketogenic diet is based on the elimination of carbohydrate-rich foods. Among these are processed foods, grains and legumes, and all sweet and starchy foods. Dairy products can also be added to the list.

PLEASE NOTE!

A hypotoxic diet is based on a gluten-free diet, without corn, without dairy products (a source of casein) and, of course, with a minimum of toxic foods to maintain or restore your health, which means eating organic foods, in season and local, if possible. Just because a food is organic doesn't mean it's automatically healthy: learn to read labels, to look for excipients, colouring, lactose, gluten, maltodextrin and starches. Opt for natural, unprocessed and unrefined foods – and always try to cook your own meals. Too many pollutants, chemical products, antibiotics and pesticides are found in our food, so boycott these for your health and your family's heath!

PROCESSED FOODS

Ready-made foods are often enriched with a wide range of additives (such as preservatives and colouring), with added sugar (to make food more appetizing and extend its shelf life), lactose, gluten, corn, starch, maltodextrin and an entire list of E numbers! Also, the quality of the fats used (hydrogenized, carcinogenic fats, for instance) often leaves a lot to be desired. And don't forget that ready-made foods, such as pizza and pasta, are often based on starches and refined grains. These are truly bad for your health and your weight!

THE ALTERNATIVES

• Cooking at home with natural, unrefined and organic foods! There are so many tips and recipes to help you quickly make your own healthy meals, which are balanced, low in carbohydrates and rich in good fats. Cook with bad fats and foods containing antibiotics and lots of toxins and you are not going to improve your health!

COOKED GRAINS & LEGUMES

High in carbohydrates, grains (such as wheat in all its forms, rice and oats) and cooked legumes (such as lentils and chickpeas) are to be avoided in a ketogenic diet.

THE ALTERNATIVES

• Instead of cooked legumes, try a small portion of sprouted legumes along with some other sprouted seeds.
• Instead of standard flour, try almond flour – it's ideal in cakes. You could also try coconut flour.
• Instead of bread, try raw crackers (with seeds and some sauerkraut) found in vegan food stores, homemade crackers rich in seeds (see page 119) and low-carb bread (see page 110).

SUGAR & SUGAR PRODUCTS

A major source of carbohydrates, sugar and sugar products (such as honey, jam and sweets) don't have a place in the ketogenic diet. There are, however, some low-GI alternatives for those who may have trouble letting go of the taste of sugar.

THE ALTERNATIVES

• Instead of powdered sugar (for sprinkling or in recipes), try a pinch of coconut sugar, a drizzle of coconut syrup or a pinch of natural organic stevia (which is green in colour). Ideally, also use spices (such as vanilla or cinnamon) or a pinch of raw cacao.

- Instead of jam or a spread, try coconut oil or unsweetened oily purees, such as almond, hazelnut, sesame, hemp or walnut.
- As a tasty snack, try a square of 100 per cent raw cacao.

AND WHAT ABOUT FRUCTOSE & AGAVE SYRUP?

Some sugars are often seen as being healthier than white sugar – but is this really the case? Fructose (fruit sugar) is a monosaccharide with a low GI, which gives it – wrongly – a good reputation. Consumed in moderation and in its natural form (with the fruit fibre), it presents no health problems. However, studies have shown that taking added fructose increases appetite, promotes weight gain and insulin resistance, produces accumulation of liver fat, metabolic syndrome, bloating, flatulence and diarrhoea, and raises triglycerides in the blood. Agave syrup has had a good press because of its low GI – but exactly the same warnings apply. Corn syrup, fruit spreads, fructose powder (jam with fructose), agave and all its derivatives should therefore be avoided and healthier alternatives used.

AND WHAT ABOUT SYNTHETIC SWEETENERS?

Aspartame and similar sweeteners are synthetic products, made using a chemical process. Some studies have suggested carcinogenic and obesity-promoting links. The body is tricked, and even though the GI of these sweeteners is zero, the body will still produce insulin. They therefore have an effect on insulin and cause weight gain. Moreover, when the body is tricked like this, you are likely to eat two to three times more food.

The most worrying thing of all, however, is the possibility of a link (although unproven) between cancer and sweeteners found in fizzy drinks and many other processed foods. The sweetener aspartame was discovered by chance in 1965 by a chemist and authorized for the first time for the United States market in 1974. But after numerous scientists revealed its toxic effect, it was banned, although then reintroduced in 1981. Other sweeteners, such as mannitol, erythritol, sorbitol, sucralose and cyclamate, are not much better. They too may have neurotoxic and carcinogenic effects. When there are natural, healthy sweeteners, why take the chance with synthetic versions?

DAIRY PRODUCTS

Because of their pro-inflammatory effect, dairy products with animal milk should be avoided. But we can opt instead for their plant-based alternatives.

DAIRY ALTERNATIVES

- Instead of yogurt, try coconut milk yogurt or a chia pudding.
- Instead of cow's milk, try plant-based milks, preferably from oily foods (such as almond, coconut, hazelnut, macadamia and sacha inchi), which you can easily make at home (see page 124).
- Instead of butter, try coconut oil, red palm oil, extra-virgin first cold pressed oils or oily butters – perfect as a spread or to cook with.
- Instead of crème fraiche, try plain coconut cream or coconut milk (other plant-based creams often contain additives).
- Instead of cheese made with cow's, goat's or sheep's milk, try plant-based cheeses. It's in fact perfectly possible to make your own cheese spreads, using macadamia nuts or cashew nuts (see page 121).

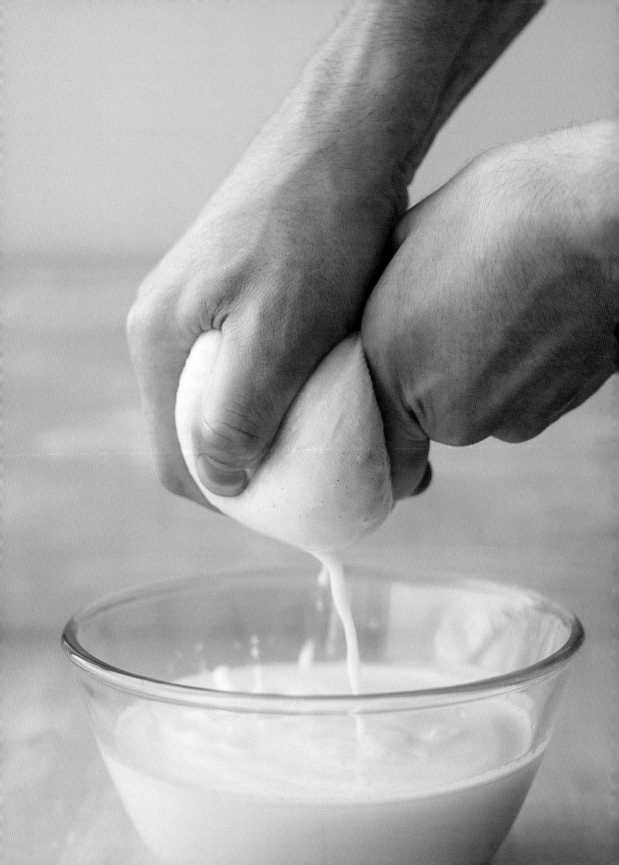

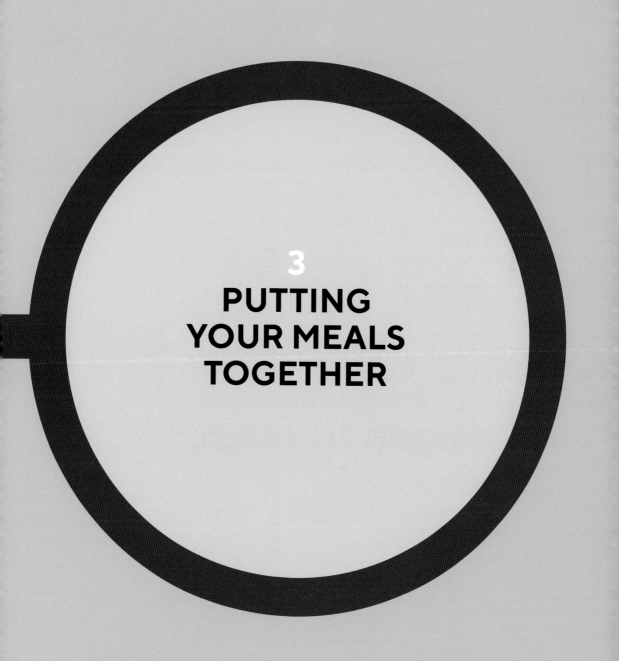

3

PUTTING YOUR MEALS TOGETHER

HOW TO MAKE A KETOGENIC BREAKFAST

Of all our daily meals, breakfast is often the one highest in carbohydrates – and first thing in the morning is the worst possible time of day to be eating carbohydrates! Breakfast should therefore be the first meal on the list to change.

NO MORE CARBOHYDRATES FOR BREAKFAST!

Whether your breakfast formula is orange juice + bread + jam + sugar or the combination of cereals + milk, you are consuming an enormous amount of carbohydrates. For example, three slices of bread (which is around 100 g) contain the equivalent of thirteen sugar cubes! A 50 g (1¾ oz) bowl of cereals rich in fibre and fruit is the equivalent of eleven sugar cubes. This excess sugar has consequences: it inevitably leads to an energy slump around 10.30–11 am with a craving for sugar, a bar of chocolate or a sweet coffee. Because sugar demands more sugar, the types of breakfast mentioned above in fact lead to high blood sugar levels, which create a feeling of tiredness and a further craving for sugar, resulting in the need for a snack to tide you over until lunchtime. This yo-yo effect can last all day and leads to excess levels of insulin in the blood. You are overworking your pancreas, and at this rate you'll be heading towards insulin resistance as well as continued weight gain.

The excessive intake of sugar in a short space of time is harmful: most of these sugars will be converted into triglycerides because their storage, in the form of glucose (in the liver and muscles), is very limited, especially if you don't exercise daily or don't have a physically demanding job! Working on a computer doesn't immediately use up the mass of carbohydrates this kind of breakfast supplies.

Simple carbohydrates create an imbalance in the intestinal microbiota to the benefit of appetite-stimulating bacteria and have a pro-inflammatory effect (leading to glucose intolerance and therefore increasing the risk of cardiovascular diseases). You get tired, you lack energy and, in the long run, your immune system also suffers. On top of that, the carbohydrate-heavy type of breakfast (including sugar, grains and juice) is extremely acidifying.

Result: a high-carbohydrate meal in the morning on an empty stomach creates a 'glycemic flash', which generates a sharp insulin spike with huge repercussions across the rest of the day.

THE ALTERNATIVES

A breakfast made with good fats and quality proteins!

- **A breakfast low in carbohydrates.**
- **Good fatty acids** (omega-3s as well as omega-9s but never too many omega-6s), including coconut oil, which will help you to produce more ketones.
- **Proteins** – we benefit most from these in the mornings as they supply tyrosine, an essential amino acid that makes dopamine, a neurotransmitter for action and energy. You can be sure of feeling full all day and know you are taking good care of yourself, both physically and mentally. This will be also reflected in increased energy, clarity and concentration.

PLEASE NOTE!

If you can't do without coffee, make sure you have no more than one coffee a day.

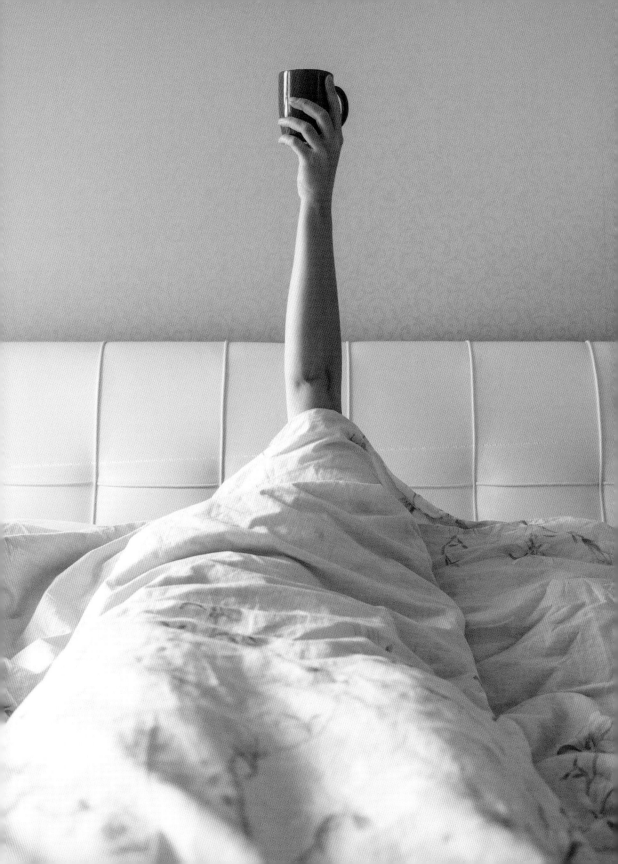

BEST FOODS FOR BREAKFAST
DRINKS
- Green tea and herbal teas such as lemon and ginger, rosemary, lemon thyme and rooibos
- Milks made from almonds, coconut, sacha inchi, sesame, hemp or macadamia (see page 124)

GOOD FATTY ACIDS
- Avocado
- Almond or hazelnut puree
- Coconut or sacha inchi oil
- Oily foods (almonds, hazelnuts, walnuts)
- Seeds (flax, chia, hemp)

PROTEINS
- Boiled eggs or a runny omelette
- Organic plant protein powder – plain, pure and, if possible, sprouted (rice, peas, hemp)
- Lacto-fermented raw cold meats (Parma ham)

HOW TO USE THESE INGREDIENTS: THE KETOGENIC PORRIDGE
- Plant-based milk (homemade, if possible)
- 1 tablespoon of plant proteins
- 2 tablespoons of organic low-carb almond flour
- 1 tablespoon of freshly ground chia seeds or homemade chia jelly (previously prepared and stored in the fridge)

PLANT POWER!
Increase the plant proteins to 2 tablespoons for athletes and vegans.

Other optional complementary ingredients (not all at the same time!):
- 1 tablespoon of freshly ground flaxseeds
- A few pinches of organic vanilla or cinnamon powder
- 1 tablespoon of raw cacao
- 1 tablespoon of organic coconut cream or 1 tablespoon of coconut oil
- 1 teaspoon of maca
- 1 teaspoon of acai
- Low-carb option (to sweeten): 1 teaspoon of raw carob + 1 tablespoon of lucuma, or 1 tablespoon of coconut syrup or kitul syrup

Prepare your porridge with more or less liquid, for a more or less creamy consistency as desired. This breakfast is very filling, and you won't be hungry before 1 pm.

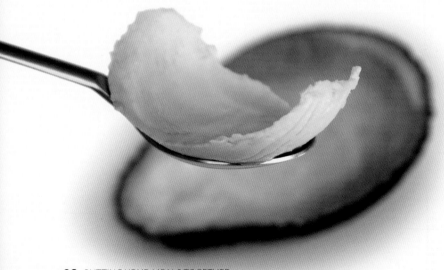

DISCOVER ... INTERMITTENT FASTING

To increase your adaptation to ketosis, you can include an intermittent fast once a week or more (even every day). In practical terms, this means not eating between 9 pm the day before and 1 pm the next day. The main thing is to keep a fasting phase of sixteen hours, which you can adapt according to your needs.

What are the health benefits of doing this while on a low-carb or ketogenic diet? Fasting in the morning is a healthy and risk-free solution. By not eating in the mornings, you extend the 'involuntary' fasting period by around eight hours (the time you spend sleeping) and enjoy all the benefits of fasting without the restrictions, risk and stress of not doing it correctly. In addition, if you want to lose weight, this can be a real boost (so long as you don't devour food at the next meal!). It's also a very good way to enter into ketosis more quickly. If you're motivated to do it and want to enjoy the benefits of the ketogenic diet more quickly, you can start with three days of intermittent fasting (by skipping breakfast).

INTERMITTENT FASTING IN PRACTICE

• Don't eat anything until 1 pm. This helps you fast every day for around sixteen hours and allows the whole of your digestive tract to rest.
• It's important to drink liquids during this fasting period. Drink a large glass of water in the morning as soon as you get up, then herbal tea, green tea or maté. Drink lots of spring water until 1 pm as well as herbal and other teas of your choice.

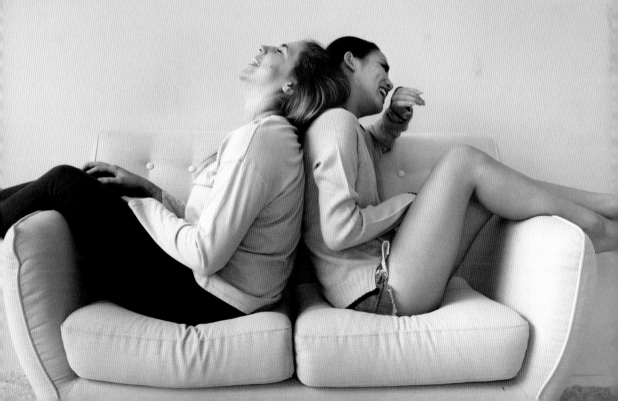

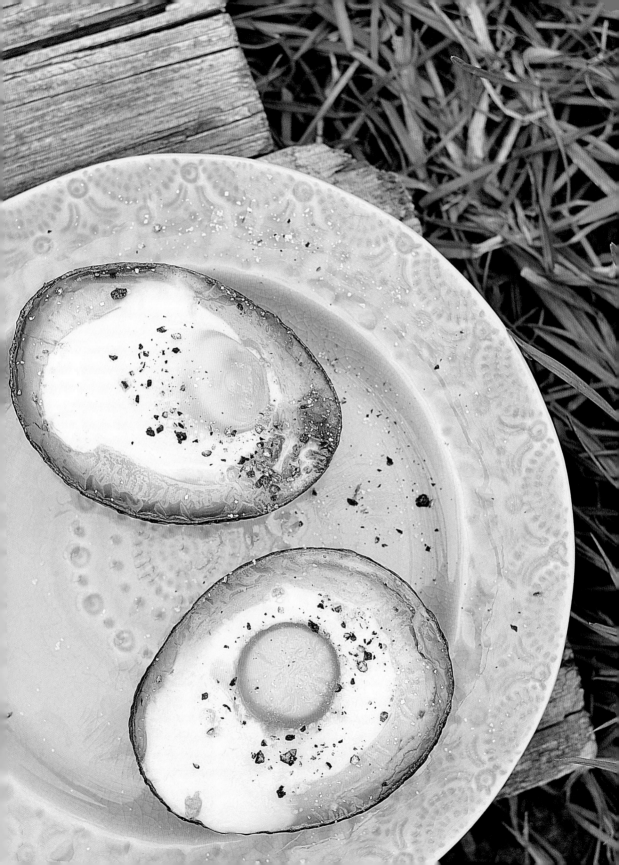

7 KETOGENIC BREAKFAST IDEAS

For a little variety, here are seven ketogenic breakfast formulas to try.

IDEA 1

EGGS-AVOCADO
- Lemon and ginger herbal tea and 1 teaspoon of coconut oil
- 2 boiled eggs
- 1 avocado + 1 teaspoon of ground flaxseeds

IDEA 2

CHIA-ALMONDS
- Maté
- Porridge with chia seeds (with homemade almond milk, sprouted rice protein, raw cacao, coconut oil and maca)

IDEA 3

CHIA-COCONUT
- Green tea
- Porridge with chia seeds (with coconut milk, pea protein, nutsedge and maca flour)

IDEA 4

EGGS-CURED HAM
- Rosemary herbal tea
- Runny omelette (2 eggs, 1 avocado, lacto-fermented cured ham, such as Parma ham), cooked with coconut oil

IDEA 5

CHIA-HEMP-ALMONDS
- Lemon thyme herbal tea
- Chia seed porridge (with almond milk, hemp protein, almond and raw cacao flour)

IDEA 6

YOGURT & AVOCADO-SPIRULINA
- Maté
- Coconut milk yogurt or chia seed yogurt with spices or cacao (see page 124)
- 1 avocado + spirulina flakes

IDEA 7

HIGH-PROTEIN MATCHA MILK
- Chia porridge (with almond milk, coconut oil, vanilla, matcha tea, maca and plant proteins)

HOW TO MAKE KETOGENIC MEALS

REDUCE YOUR INTAKE OF CARBOHYDRATES

- Avoid 'white' foods and opt instead for whole foods: wholewheat or semi-wholewheat pasta (according to your digestive tolerance), wholewheat bread, brown rice – and always organic.
- Reduce gluten and instead choose pseudo-grains such as quinoa. Avoid wheat, corn and oats, which are all high in pro-inflammatory substances, and aim for bulgur, buckwheat, quinoa and amaranth grains.
- Never eat foods highest in carbohydrates, such as pasta, bread and rice, on their own. Always serve them with fats (coconut oil, red palm oil or oily puree) and fibre (preferably green vegetables) to lower the GI of the dish. You could also add a little bit of sourness (a dash of vinegar or lemon juice).
- Make green vegetables the biggest part of your meal.
- With starches, it's better to cook them gently to avoid increasing their GI. For example, boiled potatoes are better than oven-roasted ones, cooked and cooled potatoes in a salad are better than mashed potatoes. In the same way, cooking al dente is preferable. And always avoid precooked processed foods such as '3-minute pasta' or '3-minute rice', which have a very high GI.
- Even if you can't give up all dairy products, at least cut out dairy products from cows. Limit yourself to a small portion of a goat's milk-based food with the eventual goal of cutting that out completely, too.
- Use oily flours in cakes: coconut flour, nutsedge flour, almond or hazelnut flour. They do contain carbohydrates but are also rich in fibre. In addition, they have a naturally slightly sweet taste, which compensates for the absence of sugar. You can find organic low-carb almond flour online, which, depending on the brand, has 2–4g of carbohydrates. It's a very useful alternative.
- Use spices, such as cinnamon or vanilla, to sweeten, or lemon or orange rind.

A GUIDE TO KETOGENIC COOKING

Ketogenic cooking means no more ready-made meals, replacing them instead with raw foods you prepare yourself. But don't worry: you can make tasty dishes simply and without being a top chef. All you need are good utensils and good habits!

- Get yourself a steam cooker. Use this for all foods, as it allows gentle cooking. The idea is not to exceed 100°C (212°F), to avoid denaturing the foods and instead preserve their vitamins and minerals.
- A small grinder to grind flaxseeds and chia seeds, both exceptional sources of omega-3s that you can include in your daily diet.
- Start off with simple recipes. Don't put pressure on yourself right from the beginning. The idea is to make simple, quick, tasty recipes. There are plenty of ideas to inspire you in this book.
- Always buy high-quality ingredients (organic, seasonal, local).
- Rely on herbs and spices to add flavour to all your dishes: curry powder, turmeric, ginger, cumin, cinnamon, coriander.
- Don't heat oils, as they are fragile.
- Cut out sunflower oil from your cooking and start using organic first-pressed rapeseed or camelina oil for your salads.
- Add coconut oil or coconut milk when cooking your vegetables, meats and fish.

THE PERFECT KETOGENIC STORE-CUPBOARD

A shortlist of indispensable items (organic, of course), which you should always have in your cupboard for quick and easy ketogenic cooking.

- Coconut oil
- Coconut milk
- Camelina, rapeseed, sacha inchi oils (in the fridge)
- Olive oil
- Red palm oil
- Jars of lacto-fermented olives
- Organic eggs (if you're not vegan!)
- Organic coconut flour
- Organic almond flour
- Oily butters: almonds, hazelnuts
- Oily fruits and seeds: macadamia nuts, almonds, hazelnuts, brazil nuts, walnuts
- Shelled hemp seeds
- Chia seeds
- Golden flaxseed

- Nutsedge flour
- Natural stevia
- Avocados
- Plain sauerkraut (in the winter)
- Seaweed tartare or seaweed flakes
- Low-carb vegetables in season: leeks, cabbage, courgettes, asparagus, baby lettuce, salad, endives, sprouted seeds
- Superfoods: protein powder, spirulina flakes, acai
- 100 per cent raw cacao (beans, powder, bar)
- Raw cocoa butter
- Spices: turmeric, ginger, cardamom, clove, cinnamon, vanilla, pink peppercorns, cumin
- Psyllium

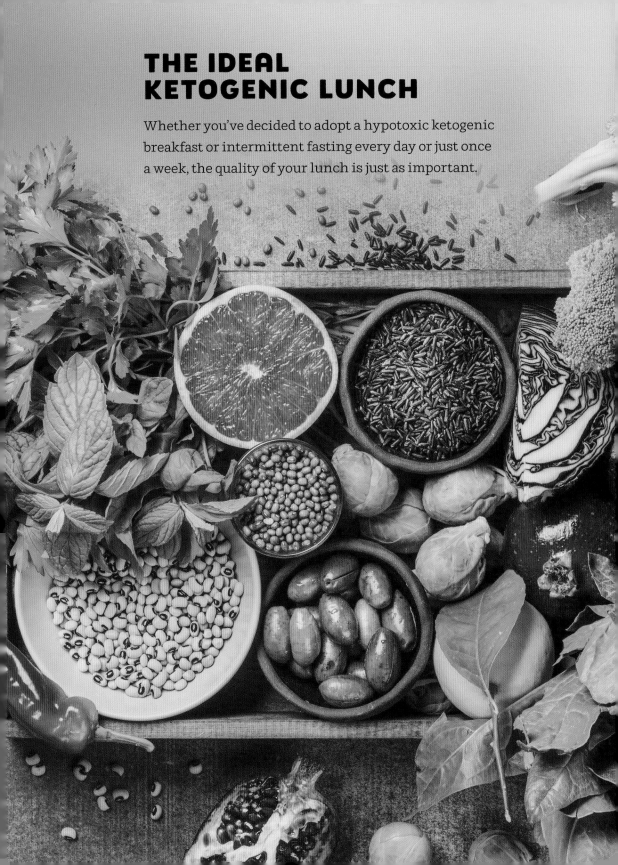

THE IDEAL
KETOGENIC LUNCH

Whether you've decided to adopt a hypotoxic ketogenic breakfast or intermittent fasting every day or just once a week, the quality of your lunch is just as important.

9 KETOGENIC LUNCH IDEAS

For a little variety, here are nine ketogenic lunch formulas to try.

IDEA 1

DUCK CONFIT AND 'RICE'
- Grated black radish with camelina oil
- Duck leg confit
- Cauliflower 'rice' (see page 114)

IDEA 2

CHICKEN-LEEKS
- Organic chicken fillet or thigh
- Leek fondue made with red palm oil

IDEA 3

MIXED SALAD
- Salad made with endives, walnuts, pine nuts, avocado and cured ham

IDEA 4

SEAFOOD MENU
- Sardines or scallop carpaccio
- Salad made with lamb's lettuce, rocket, sprouted seeds, ground flaxseeds, flakes or chips of oily fruit and seeds, camelina and olive oils

IDEA 5

VEGETARIAN LUNCH
- Broccoli steamed in coconut milk, sesame puree and poached eggs

IDEA 6

VEGAN LUNCH (LIVING FOODS)
- Sauerkraut (raw) and camelina oil
- Avocado and lacto-fermented tofu with olives

IDEA 7

VEGAN LUNCH (LIVING FOODS)
- Avocado pesto with acai (see page 121)
- Baby leaf salad (spinach, rocket, lamb's lettuce) with pumpkin seeds, chia and shelled hemp seeds

IDEA 8

VEGAN SPAGHETTI BOLOGNAISE (LIVING FOODS)
- Courgette spaghetti in tomato sauce with vegetable patties (see page 113)

IDEA 9

VEGAN PIZZA (LIVING FOODS)
- Keto-pizza (see page 117)

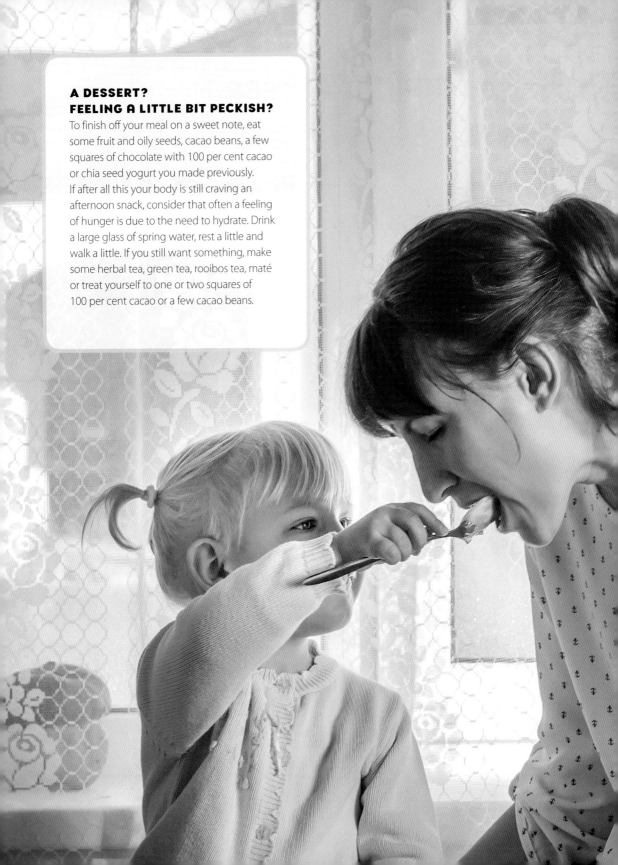

A DESSERT?
FEELING A LITTLE BIT PECKISH?

To finish off your meal on a sweet note, eat some fruit and oily seeds, cacao beans, a few squares of chocolate with 100 per cent cacao or chia seed yogurt you made previously.

If after all this your body is still craving an afternoon snack, consider that often a feeling of hunger is due to the need to hydrate. Drink a large glass of spring water, rest a little and walk a little. If you still want something, make some herbal tea, green tea, rooibos tea, maté or treat yourself to one or two squares of 100 per cent cacao or a few cacao beans.

THE KETOGENIC DINNER

Whenever we run out of time in the evenings, it's often tempting to go for the simplest solution: get a pizza delivered, cook some pasta or put a ready-made meal in the microwave. So how about taking dinner back into your own hands?

In fact, it's easy and quick to prepare very good soups, raw or cooked. And never forget, it's always the quality of the food you choose that makes the difference in taste. You could also prepare raw salads such as grated black radish, which also happens to be excellent for your liver, with some camelina or sacha inchi oil.

It isn't always necessary to eat meat in the evenings, and it may even be preferable to avoid it, especially when you are in need of restorative sleep. Dinner could then be made of vegetables and good fats and occasionally, if you like, eggs and a very small portion of sprouted fruit and seeds. Your two main basic evening meals from now on: keto-adapted soups and keto-adapted raw salads.

KETO-ADAPTED SOUPS, A HOW-TO GUIDE

What's the secret to converting a standard soup into a ketogenic and hypotoxic soup? Cut out the starch (such as potatoes, squash or sweet potato) and replace crème fraiche or butter with coconut milk.

- Opt for leeks and cabbages (such as green cabbage or savoy cabbage). In fact, the two combined are delicious. And why not add in a small carrot or a little turnip? This won't take you out of ketosis if you've been following a keto-adapted diet all day.
- Freeze your vegetables (such as courgettes, broccoli, cauliflower and fennel). When you don't have the time to shop for organic, seasonal and local vegetables, always keep a small stock of these.
- To thicken your soup, add 1 tablespoon of psyllium or a little chia jelly, pre-prepared and stored in your fridge. Or try some shelled hemp seeds.
- Rely on spices: one clove, two pink peppercorns and two juniper berries in your soup's cooking water. These spices are high in antioxidants and have many health properties.

- To flavour your soup and enrich it with probiotics that are good for your intestinal flora, you can add ¼ teaspoon of organic unpasteurized rice miso. Be careful to add this directly into your bowl – and don't boil it or salt it as miso is already salted.
- Avoid tap water (boiling it will not alter its endocrine disruptor content).

SOUP ... OR SIMPLY SOME STEAMED VEGETABLES!

As a change from soups, also think about vegetables that are simply steam cooked. Then add in some olive oil or coconut oil – or red palm oil, which will change their colour – as well as spices (such as turmeric, cumin, cardamom, ginger and cayenne pepper). A quick and delicious meal!

KETO-ADAPTED RAW SALADS

- Low-carbohydrate vegetables: black radish or daikon radish combined with camelina oil, a little umeboshi vinegar (or a drizzle of lemon juice) and a few shelled hemp seeds. A salad rich in phytonutrients and omega-3s!
- To serve with your raw salads (such as pink radish, celery sticks or cauliflower heads), rely on ketogenic dips that are delicious and quick to prepare.
- Tabbouleh-style cauliflower semolina is also quick to prepare.
- Raw vegetables in the form of spaghetti or tagliatelle, angel hair or spiralized.
- Lacto-fermented vegetables that you've prepared yourself a few weeks in advance. Always have these in stock! You can also buy plain sauerkraut (with only salt and no white wine or other ingredients) from the fresh produce section at an organic store. Feel free to eat a little every day – it's perfect for restoring the balance of our microbiota.

7 KETOGENIC DINNER IDEAS

For a little variety, here are seven ketogenic dinner formulas to try.

IDEA 1

DIP AND SOUP
- Avocado pesto (see page 121) and raw vegetable sticks (such as celery, radish, cucumber or endives) or crackers (see page 119)
- Cooked cauliflower soup (see page 107)
- Coconut milk yogurt

IDEA 2

TAPENADE AND SOUP
- Black olive and avocado tapenade and raw vegetable sticks (such as celery, radish, cucumber or endives)
- Savoy cabbage and leek soup (see page 107)
- Pieces of fresh coconut

IDEA 3

GUACAMOLE AND BROCCOLI
- Guacamole
- Rocket and sprouted seeds salad, camelina oil
- Broccoli with coconut milk and sesame paste (see page 115)
- Herbal tea and cacao beans

IDEA 4

VEGETABLES AND PUREE
- Lacto-fermented vegetables, olives and camelina oil
- Cauliflower and coconut puree (see page 114)
- Chia seed yogurt with spices (see page 124)

IDEA 5

SPINACH AND SOUP
- Cooked cauliflower soup (see page 107)
- Spinach with coconut oil
- Chia seed yogurt with spices (see page 124)

IDEA 6

AVOCADO AND COURGETTES STIR-FRY
- Avocado, spirulina twigs and black olives
- Courgettes with red palm oil
- Coconut milk yogurt

IDEA 7

GAZPACHO AND CHEESE
- Gazpacho
- Macadamia nut cheese (see page 121) and raw vegetable sticks (such as celery, radish, cucumber or endives)
- Avocado, almond milk, cinnamon and vanilla milkshake

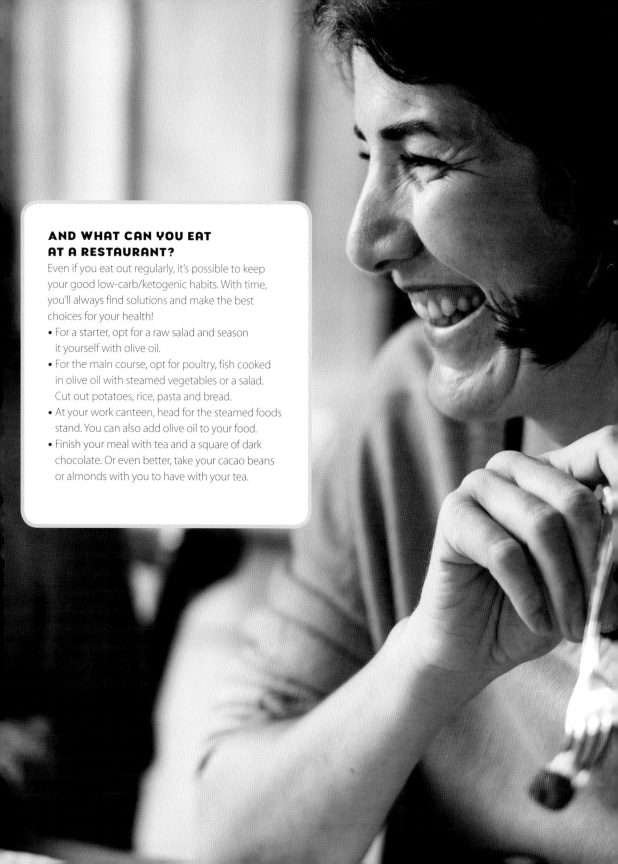

AND WHAT CAN YOU EAT AT A RESTAURANT?

Even if you eat out regularly, it's possible to keep your good low-carb/ketogenic habits. With time, you'll always find solutions and make the best choices for your health!

- For a starter, opt for a raw salad and season it yourself with olive oil.
- For the main course, opt for poultry, fish cooked in olive oil with steamed vegetables or a salad. Cut out potatoes, rice, pasta and bread.
- At your work canteen, head for the steamed foods stand. You can also add olive oil to your food.
- Finish your meal with tea and a square of dark chocolate. Or even better, take your cacao beans or almonds with you to have with your tea.

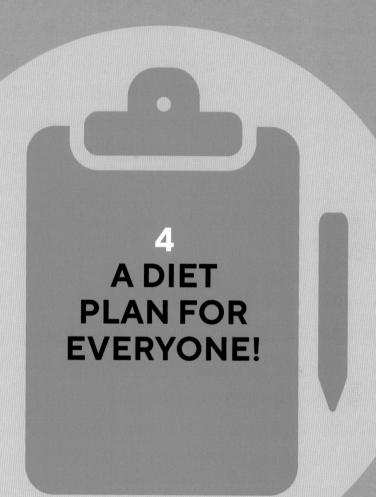

4
**A DIET
PLAN FOR
EVERYONE!**

Now that you know the
fundamentals of the ketogenic diet, you may
want to adopt a ketogenic and hypotoxic diet
according to specific goals, a health issue or for a more
balanced vegetarian or vegan diet plan.

HERE ARE THREE WEEK-LONG PLANS:
- The weight-loss plan
- The anti-inflammatory plan, to fight cancer, autoimmune and neurodegenerative diseases
- The vegetarian/vegan plan

FOR EACH OF THESE PLANS, YOU WILL FIND:
- An explanation of the goal to be achieved
- Some practical advice on starting the plan and ensuring its success, according to your goals
- Weekly menus, some of which include detailed recipes in the recipe section, as well as the corresponding shopping list for that week of the plan

HOW TO START A KETOGENIC & HYPOTOXIC DIET

Before introducing you to these three plans, let's first take a look at the required stages leading up to a ketogenic diet. In fact, these are so contrary to the usual recommendations, and to some food habits, that putting it all into practice can seem difficult, even overwhelming.

Cutting out most carbohydrates from your diet overnight – suddenly giving up bread, pasta and sugar as well as your usual bread–jam–juice breakfast – can feel like fighting a losing battle. Naturally, this will depend on your motivation, willpower and, most of all, the initial state of your health. It's still possible to make the change in one go, but it's better to do it in stages. If necessary, you could engage a therapist specialized in ketogenic and hypotoxic diets to guide you on a daily basis with this radical change.

On a more practical level, before taking the plunge, you'll need to go through a preparatory phase, both physical and mental. In fact, you must want to take care of yourself and your body and be fully aware of this. The transition phase to a truly ketogenic diet generally takes six weeks.

FOUR RECOMMENDATIONS FOR STARTING THE PROCESS

1. IDENTIFY THE SUGARS AND CARBOHYDRATES YOU CONSUME AT EACH OF YOUR MEALS

AS A REMINDER, THEY ARE FOUND IN:

- **sweet foods** (such as honey, jam, fizzy drinks, sweets and chocolate)
- **fruit**
- **dairy products**
- **grains and grain products** (such as bread, pasta, biscuits, pastries and pizzas)
- **pseudo-grains** (such as quinoa, buckwheat, amaranth and fonio)
- **nonsprouted legumes** (such as lentils and chickpeas)
- **tubers** (such as potato, sweet potato, yam, cassava and plantain banana)
- **squashes** (such as winter squash, squash and butternut squash)
- **root vegetables** (such as parsnip and sweet potato)
- **processed foods**, even in products theoretically categorized as salty, such as sauces or processed soups; their sweetening additives have names like 'glucose syrup', 'glucose/fructose', 'corn syrup', 'maltodextrin' or 'lactose'

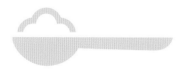

2. CHOOSE FOODS THAT ARE LOWER IN CARBOHYDRATES

- **Avoid 'white' foods** (always opt for whole or semi-whole foods): wholewheat bread rather than white bread, for example, or wholewheat pasta instead of white pasta.
- **Choose oily flours instead of grain-based flours** (such as coconut flour, almond flour, nutsedge flour and hazelnut flour).
- **Sweeten foods with spices or citrus peel.**
- **Always combine high-carbohydrate foods** (such as pasta, bread and rice) **with a fat source** (such as coconut oil, red palm oil and oily puree).
- **With starches, opt for gently cooked foods to prevent a rise in the GI.** For example, choose potatoes boiled in water rather than roasted in an oven, cold cooked potatoes in a salad rather than mashed potato. Similarly, opt for al dente cooking. Always avoid precooked processed foods such as '3-minute pasta' or '3-minute rice', which have a very high GI.
- **Even if you can't give up all dairy products, at least cut out dairy products from cows.** Limit yourself to a small portion of a goat's milk-based food, with the eventual goal of cutting this out completely too.

3. ADOPT NEW SHOPPING AND COOKING HABITS

(see also 'The perfect ketogenic store-cupboard' on page 73)

- **Choose good-quality raw foods** (organic, local and seasonal) and steer clear of ready-made processed foods.
- **Read labels to avoid sugars, carbohydrates, excipients and colourants.**
- **Get yourself a steam cooker.**
- **Use aromatic herbs and spices to flavour your dishes.**
- **Cut out sunflower oil from your cooking** and start using organic first-pressed rapeseed or camelina oil for your salads. Add coconut oil or coconut milk when cooking your vegetables, meats and fish.
- **Opt for small oily fish**, such as sardines, anchovies and mackerel, for their high omega-3 levels and low mercury levels.

4. GRADUALLY START CHANGING YOUR BREAKFAST, LUNCH AND DINNER CHOICES

(following the recommendations provided in the previous chapter)

Over the weeks, you'll notice clear changes in your shape, the state of your digestive tract, your weight, inflammatory issues and, if applicable, your muscle mass, stress levels, athletic performance and more. Seeing these positive changes will boost your motivation and make transitioning to a ketogenic and hypotoxic diet so much easier.

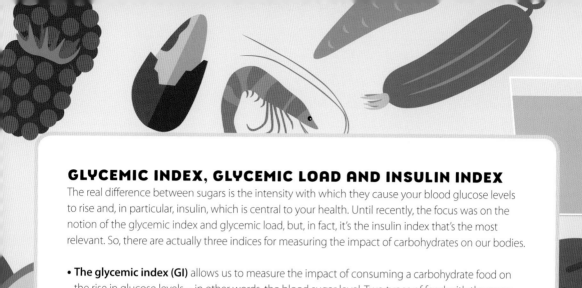

GLYCEMIC INDEX, GLYCEMIC LOAD AND INSULIN INDEX

The real difference between sugars is the intensity with which they cause your blood glucose levels to rise and, in particular, insulin, which is central to your health. Until recently, the focus was on the notion of the glycemic index and glycemic load, but, in fact, it's the insulin index that's the most relevant. So, there are actually three indices for measuring the impact of carbohydrates on our bodies.

- **The glycemic index (GI)** allows us to measure the impact of consuming a carbohydrate food on the rise in glucose levels – in other words, the blood sugar level. Two types of food with the same carbohydrate level could therefore have totally different effects on our glucose levels. The higher the GI, the greater the rise in blood sugar levels. The value 0 corresponds to that of water, the value 100 corresponds to that of glucose (pure sugar). On this scale, we generally distinguish between foods with a low GI (less than 55), a medium GI (between 56 and 69) and a high GI (more than 70).

- **The glycemic load (GL)** also takes into account the notion of portion size of the food ingested, its fibre and water content, and the quantity. The notion of glycemic load allows us to evaluate a food's capacity to raise our glucose levels for a typical portion size. It's simple to calculate – just multiply the GI by the amount of carbohydrates contained in a typical portion size and divide the total by 100. On this scale, we generally distinguish between foods with a low GL (less than 10 – a serving of tinned peas, for example) and foods with a high GL (more than 20 – a serving of cooked white rice, for example). This allows us to be more precise on the impact of the portion size ingested on our glucose levels, while also taking into account the quantity.

- **The insulin index (II)** measures the insulin released following the intake of a particular food (as a reminder, insulin is the hormone produced by the pancreas, which allows sugar to enter the cells). The baseline insulin index is that of white bread, which is 100, while that of confectionary such as chocolate bars or sweets is 160. For very many foods, the GIs and IIs are correlated. However, some foods can have a low GI but a high II. This is the case for dairy products containing whey (such as plain yogurt or cheese). For example, a plain yogurt has a GI of 62 and an II of 115 (more than white bread and the equivalent of a chocolate bar). Adding milk, even in small quantities, to a food also increases the insulin index of the food ingested. This is therefore the most important calculation to be taken into account.

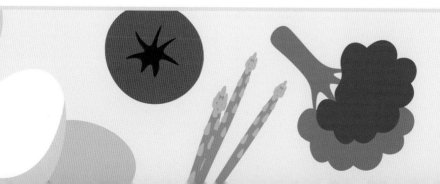

THE WEIGHT-LOSS PLAN

Are you trying to lose weight? The goal is to set up a diet during this starting period, which, once you have reached your target weight, can be a little less ketogenic and a little less low carb. But the basic principles will remain the same.

You should avoid losing weight too rapidly. Our fats store all the toxins that our liver cannot get rid of. When these fats are eliminated, the liver has to take on the job of releasing these toxins into the blood circulation. It's therefore healthier, depending on the amount of weight you wish to lose, to spread this initial diet stage over several weeks or months and to fix a goal – six months, for example.

PLEASE NOTE!
- Feel free to get advice from a nutritional therapist or naturopath trained in ketogenic nutrition to guide you during your dietary changes.
- The high nutritional value of the foods consumed is vital. In fact, with this plan, the quantity of food is reduced, and all foods lacking nutritional value – which are also fatiguing – are cut out.
- Depending on your medical condition, it's important to talk to your doctor to check certain biological markers, especially if you take any medications. Your glucose and insulin levels will fall sharply, which will have a positive impact on your health, but your prescription doses will almost certainly have to be changed.

To support your liver function, you could follow a treatment course using milk thistle or desmodium – both plants with detoxing properties. Several times a week, as a supplement to this treatment, you could also eat detoxifying bitter plants such as black radish, raw endives or dandelions.

ANOTHER IDEA

Try a birch sap treatment course over three weeks in the spring. Take this in the mornings or at noon on an empty stomach to drain and help the body with the elimination of toxins.

HOW TO FOLLOW THE PLAN

- Before starting the plan, first measure your waist and hips.
- Weigh yourself when you have an empty stomach and note the percentage of lean body mass and fat mass (with biometric weighing scales). Measure weight and lean and fat mass over three consecutive days and calculate the average. This will give you more accurate numbers. After that, you can take the same measurements once a week or even every two weeks. Note all measurements down in a notebook.
- Start the plan with an intermittent fast of at least three days to enter into ketosis (first meal of the day at 1 pm, last meal before 9 pm). If you are still not in ketosis, continue with the intermittent fast: there are no risks if you stick to the dietary recommendations. Include two intermittent fasts during the plan week – for example, on Monday and Wednesday. You can do the intermittent fast whenever you find your weight is stagnating to burn more fats.
- If possible, start doing some physical exercise on an empty stomach twice a week in the mornings (for example, on Monday and Wednesday) for around 30–45 minutes. If you don't have a lot of time, keep it to 15–20 minutes.
- Remember to be as active as possible during the day: take long walks and get some fresh air in the woods at the weekend (Nordic walking is the perfect activity to work all the muscles of the body).

PACE YOURSELF!

If you haven't done any kind of physical exercise in a long while, go gradually. It's more important to be moderately active every day rather than plan one big session once a week.

- Keep a food diary to note down what you eat and track your progress as you change your diet. Eventually this will no longer be necessary as you will have adopted new long-lasting habits.
- Use test strips to check your state of ketosis every morning on an empty stomach. You'll see if you have slightly deviated straightaway. It's easy to move out of ketosis quickly.
- Don't forget to reward yourself for all your efforts towards a new lifestyle that is healthy for every cell in your body. This could mean a massage or shiatsu session – you can treat yourself in so many ways other than with cakes or biscuits!

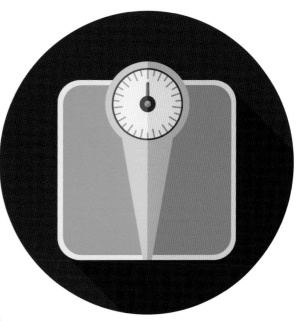

MENUS FOR THE WEEK

This is your menu plan for the week. Start this after three days of intermittent fasting.

MONDAY

On waking up Spring water

Breakfast intermittent fast

Throughout the morning
Maté, herbal tea (rosemary, thyme or lemon and ginger) + spring water

Lunch
- 1 large glass of spring water
- 2 slices of cured ham
- Endive salad (with 1 tbsp of camelina oil, walnut pieces and hemp seeds)
- 1 avocado
- 1 or 2 squares of 100 per cent dark chocolate
- 1 cinnamon tea (1 cinnamon stick infused for 10 minutes in 200 ml/7 fl oz of boiling spring water)

During the afternoon
Green tea, maté, herbal tea (rosemary, thyme or lemon and ginger) + spring water

Dinner
- 1 runny omelette (2 eggs + 1 tbsp of coconut oil)
- Grated green or white cabbage (with 1 tbsp of camelina oil, walnut pieces and hemp seeds)
- 1 chia seed yogurt with spices (see page 124)
- 1 verbena herbal tea

TIP TO PREVENT SNACKING OR TO CALM YOUR HUNGER

Are you starting to feel a little peckish? Take a walk for 5–10 minutes, then drink a large glass of water or cup of herbal tea. You'll then be able to hold on until dinner.

If you're too hungry, take a handful of almonds, hazelnuts or macadamia nuts, or even black olives, with a glass of water and a slice of lemon, while cooking your meal.

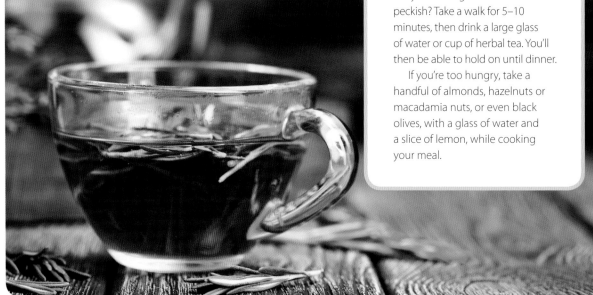

TUESDAY

On waking up Spring water

Breakfast
- Maté, herbal tea (rosemary, thyme or lemon and ginger) + spring water throughout the morning
- Almond porridge (almond milk, hemp protein, almond flour, maca, vanilla and cinnamon)

Throughout the morning
Maté, herbal tea (rosemary, thyme or lemon and ginger) + spring water

Lunch
- 1 large glass of spring water
- 3 sardines in oil
- 1 avocado
- Rocket and sprouted seeds salad (with 1 tbsp of camelina oil, walnut pieces and hemp seeds)
- 1 square of 100 per cent dark chocolate
- 1 cinnamon tea

During the afternoon
Green tea, maté, herbal tea (rosemary, thyme or lemon and ginger) + spring water

Dinner
- Vegetable soup (leeks, cabbage and spices) + 1 tsp to 1 tbsp of psyllium
- 1 chia seed yogurt with cacao (see page 124)
- 1 lemon balm tea (2–4 tsp of leaves infused in one cup of hot water for 10 minutes)

WEDNESDAY

On waking up Spring water

Breakfast intermittent fast

Throughout the morning
Maté, herbal tea (rosemary, thyme or lemon and ginger) + spring water

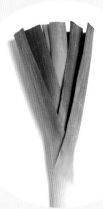

Lunch
- 1 large glass of spring water
- Duck breast
- Grated black radish salad (with 1 tbsp of sacha inchi oil and hemp seeds)
- 1 coconut milk yogurt + 1 pinch of powdered cinnamon
- 1 ginger tea (1 small piece of fresh ginger infused for 10 minutes in boiling water)

During the afternoon
Green tea, maté, herbal tea (rosemary, thyme or lemon and ginger) + spring water

Dinner
- Leek pancakes (see page 116)
- Baby spinach and lacto-fermented vegetable salad (with 1 tbsp of sacha inchi oil and 1 tsp of ume plum vinegar)
- 1 cinnamon tea

THURSDAY

On waking up Spring water

Breakfast
- Sacha inchi porridge (sacha inchi milk, plain rice protein, almond flour, maca, vanilla and cinnamon)
- Maté, herbal tea (rosemary, thyme or lemon and ginger) + spring water

Throughout the morning
Maté, herbal tea (rosemary, thyme or lemon and ginger) + spring water

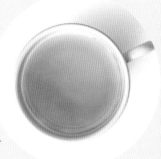

Lunch
- 1 large glass of spring water
- 150 g (5 oz) sliced turkey, steam cooked
- Cauliflower semolina, sautéed in coconut oil + 1 tsp of curry powder
- 1 avocado-cacao mousse (see page 122)
- 1 rosemary tea

During the afternoon
Green tea, maté, herbal tea (rosemary, thyme or lemon and ginger) + spring water

Dinner
- Sesame and miso broth + 1 tsp to 1 tbsp of psyllium
- 1 chia seed yogurt with with cacao (see page 124)
- 1 camomile tea

FRIDAY

On waking up Spring water

Breakfast
- 1 or 2 avocados
- 2 boiled eggs
- 1 handful of almonds (optional)
- Maté, herbal tea (rosemary, thyme or lemon and ginger) + spring water

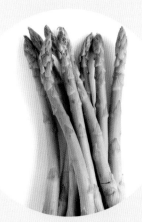

Throughout the morning
Maté, herbal tea (rosemary, thyme or lemon and ginger) + spring water

Lunch
- 1 large glass of spring water
- 3 mackerel fillets in oil from a jar (or fresh, steam cooked with lemon)
- Leek fondue (with 1 tbsp of coconut oil and 1 tsp of any spices of your choice)
- 1 square of 100 per cent dark chocolate
- 1 cinnamon tea

During the afternoon
Green tea, maté, herbal tea (rosemary, thyme or lemon and ginger) + spring water

Dinner
- Creamed asparagus + 1 tsp of psyllium
- 1 chia seed yogurt with cacao (see page 124)
- 1 anise and fennel tea

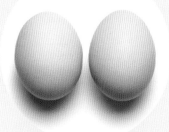

SATURDAY

On waking up Spring water

Breakfast
- Pancake with an almond–cinnamon coulis
- Maté, herbal tea (rosemary, thyme or lemon and ginger) + spring water

Throughout the morning
Maté, herbal tea (rosemary, thyme or lemon and ginger) + spring water

Lunch
- 1 large glass of spring water
- 3 sardines in oil
- Rocket and sprouted seeds salad of your choice
  (with 1 tbsp of camelina oil, walnut pieces and hemp seeds)
- 1 avocado
- 1 square of 100 per cent dark chocolate or a few cacao beans
- 1 cinnamon tea

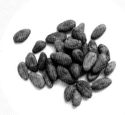

During the afternoon
Green tea, maté, herbal tea (rosemary, thyme or lemon and ginger) + spring water

Dinner
- Lacto-fermented vegetable salad (sauerkraut, for example) with 1 tbsp of camelina oil
- Macadamia nut cheese (see page 121) + cucumber, courgette and radish sticks
- Crackers (see page 119) and sprouted seeds salad of your choice (with 1 tbsp of olive oil)
- 1 lemon balm tea

SUNDAY

On waking up Spring water

Breakfast
- Almond crepes (see page 122)
- 2 slices of cured ham
- Maté, herbal tea (rosemary, thyme or lemon and ginger) + spring water

Throughout the morning
Maté, herbal tea (rosemary, thyme or lemon and ginger) + spring water

Lunch
- 1 large glass of spring water
- Raw courgette carpaccio and sacha inchi seeds
- Anchovies marinated in lemon + a few olives
- 1 coconut flan
- 1 cinnamon tea

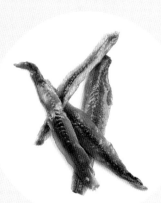

During the afternoon
Green tea, maté, herbal tea (rosemary, thyme or lemon and ginger) + spring water

Dinner
- Avocado-cashew nut soup (see page 106) + 1 tsp of psyllium
- 1 chia seed yogurt with cacao (see page 124)
- 1 verbena tea

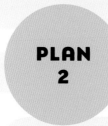

PLAN 2

THE ANTI-INFLAMMATORY PLAN

A plan that helps to fight cancer, autoimmune and neurodegenerative diseases. The harmful effects of gluten, casein, sugar and carbohydrates in general make choosing a ketogenic diet relevant to all inflammatory diseases.

A number of studies, carried out mainly in the United States, suggest that this type of diet may help in the fight against diseases such as cancer and autoimmune and neurodegenerative diseases.

HOW TO FOLLOW THE PLAN

- Begin with an intermittent fast of at least three days to enter into ketosis (first meal of the day around 1 pm, last meal before 9 pm). If you are still not in ketosis, continue the intermittent fast: there are no risks if you stick to the dietary recommendations.
- If possible, start doing some physical exercise on an empty stomach twice a week in the mornings (for example, on Monday and Wednesday) for around 30–45 minutes. If you don't have a lot of time, keep it to 15–20 minutes.

PLEASE NOTE!

- You might want to get advice from a nutritional therapist or naturopath trained in ketogenic nutrition to guide you during your dietary changes.
- Depending on your medical condition, talk to your doctor about this plan to check certain biological markers, especially if you take any medications, as your prescription doses will almost certainly have to be changed.

PLEASE NOTE!

Fasting is not obligatory. If you are anaemic and/or underweight, don't do the intermittent fast for the moment and go straight on to the weekly plan. You'll have a greater need for nutritional guidance in this case so that you can make up for deficiencies with food supplements adapted specifically to your condition.

- Remember to be as active as possible during the day. Take long walks and get some fresh air in the woods at the weekend (Nordic walking is the perfect activity to work all the muscles of the body).
- Use test strips to check your state of ketosis every morning on an empty stomach. You'll see if you have slightly deviated straightaway.
- In this plan, omega-3s are emphasized and should be eaten at each meal as well as coconut oil for its medium-chain triglycerides (MCTs). In the case of neurodegenerative disease, you should also look at organic oils rich in MCTs. Lacto-fermented vegetables should be consumed in small portions every day – for example, 1 tablespoon of sauerkraut with camelina oil as a starter each evening. The goal is to restore the balance of our microbiota.

MENUS FOR THE WEEK

Here is a typical weekly diet to follow in the case of an inflammatory disease. You should adapt these menus according to any food intolerances you may have.

MONDAY

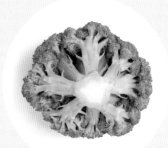

On waking up Spring water

Breakfast
- Almond porridge (almond milk, ground chia and flaxseeds, hemp protein and raw cacao – optional)
- 1 lemon and ginger herbal tea

Throughout the morning
Maté, herbal tea (rosemary, thyme or lemon and ginger) + spring water

Lunch
- 1 large glass of spring water
- Anchovies marinated in lemon
- 1 avocado
- Baby spinach, sprouted seeds and olive salad (with 1 tbsp of camelina oil and hemp seeds)
- 1 square of 100 per cent dark chocolate or a few cacao beans
- 1 ginger tea

During the afternoon
Green tea, maté, herbal tea (rooibos, rosemary, thyme or hibiscus) + spring water

Dinner
- Grated black radish salad (with 1 tbsp of camelina oil and hemp seeds)
- Steamed broccoli with spices + coconut butter with fresh turmeric and ginger (see page 117)
- 1 chia seed yogurt with spices (see page 124)
- 1 cinnamon tea

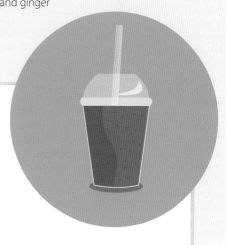

A WEAKENED NERVOUS SYSTEM?
If you have problems affecting your nervous system, you can add 1 tablespoon of an organic oil rich in MCTs to your morning smoothie or porridge, or simply to your hot drink.

Also consider fresh vegetable juice (without fruit) to fill up on minerals, vitamins and enzymes, which should be taken 30 minutes before meals. For example, 1 or 2 fennel bulbs, ½ lemon, a small piece of ginger (less than 1 cm), diluted with spring water.

TUESDAY

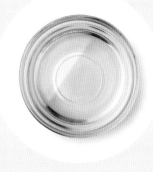

On waking up Spring water

Breakfast
- Sacha inchi smoothie (sacha inchi milk, coconut flour + ground chia seeds and flaxseeds, 1 to 2 tbsp of rice proteins and maca)
- 1 ginger tea

Throughout the morning
Maté, herbal tea (rosemary, thyme or lemon and ginger) + spring water

Lunch
- 1 large glass of spring water
- Sardines in oil
- Lacto-fermented vegetable salad (cabbage, leek and a few carrots) with 1 tsp of camelina oil and 1 tsp of olive oil
- 1 coconut milk yogurt + raw cacao and hazelnut nibs
- 1 ginger tea

During the afternoon
Green tea, maté, herbal tea (rooibos, rosemary, thyme or hibiscus) + spring water

Dinner
- Sesame–miso broth
- Steamed leek fondue with spices + coconut butter with fresh turmeric and ginger (see page 117)
- 1 chia seed yogurt with spices (see page 124)
- 1 verbena tea

WEDNESDAY

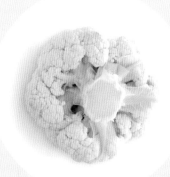

On waking up Spring water

Breakfast
- Golden turmeric milk (see page 125)
- 1 avocado
- 2 boiled eggs

Throughout the morning
Maté, herbal tea (rosemary, thyme or lemon and ginger) + spring water

Lunch
- 1 large glass of spring water
- Duck confit leg
- Cauliflower and coconut puree (see page 114) + ½ tsp of turmeric
- 1 square of 100 per cent dark chocolate or a few cacao beans
- 1 ginger tea

During the afternoon
Green tea, maté, herbal tea (rooibos, rosemary, thyme or hibiscus) + spring water

Dinner
- Avocado-cashew nut soup (see page 106)
- Almond flan
- 1 liquorice tea (except in cases of hypertension)

THURSDAY

On waking up Spring water

Breakfast
- Sacha inchi smoothie (sacha inchi milk, coconut flour +
  ground chia seeds and flaxseeds, pea proteins and raw cacao – optional)
- Maté

Throughout the morning
Maté, herbal tea (rosemary, thyme or lemon and ginger) + spring water

Lunch
- 1 large glass of spring water
- 2 or 3 slices of cured ham
- Sprouted seeds, rocket, lamb's lettuce and black olive salad (with 1 tbsp of camelina oil)
- Avocado-cacao mousse (see page 122)
- 1 ginger tea

During the afternoon
Rooibos tea + spring water

Dinner
- Lacto-fermented vegetable salad (with 1 tbsp of sacha inchi oil)
- Creamy spinach soup (see page 106)
- A few cacao beans
- 1 cinnamon tea

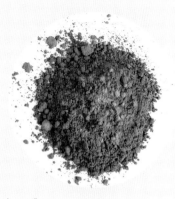

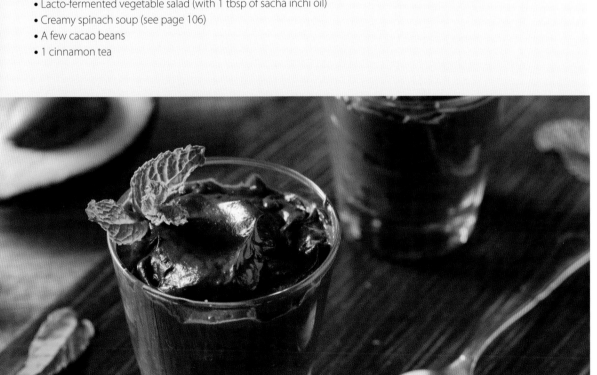

FRIDAY

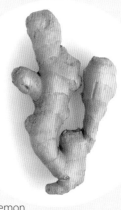

On waking up Spring waterr

Breakfast
- Pancakes with almond–coconut coulis
- 1 lemon and ginger herbal tea

Throughout the morning
Maté, herbal tea (rosemary, thyme or lemon and ginger) + spring water

Lunch
- 1 large glass of spring water
- 3 mackerel fillets in olive oil (glass jar) or fresh and steam cooked, with herbs and lemon
- Sprouted seeds and olive salad (with 1 tbsp of camelina oil)
- Courgette spaghetti with pesto
- 1 square of 100 per cent dark chocolate or a few cacao beans
- 1 ginger tea

During the afternoon
Hibiscus tea + spring water

Dinner
- Runny omelette with shiitake mushrooms (2 eggs, with 1 tbsp of coconut oil)
- Baby spinach salad (with 1 tbsp of camelina oil)
- Macadamia nut cheese (see page 121) and sauerkraut crackers (see page 119)
- 1 liquorice tea (except in cases of hypertension)

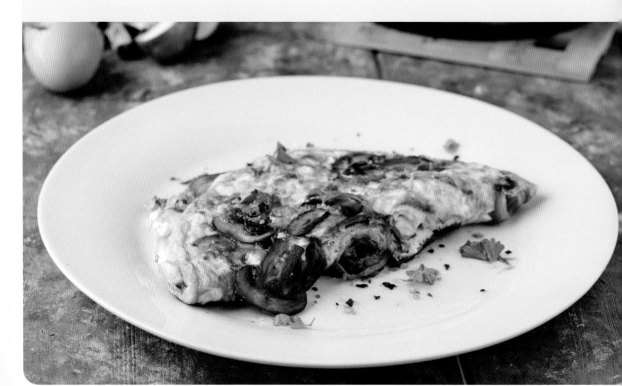

SATURDAY

On waking up Spring water

Breakfast:
- Chia seed smoothie (almond milk, ground chia seeds and flaxseeds, rice proteins, raw cacao and cinnamon)
- 1 lemon and ginger herbal tea

Throughout the morning
Maté, herbal tea (rosemary, thyme or lemon and ginger) + spring water

Lunch
- 1 large glass of spring water
- Steamed asparagus
- 3 slices of cured ham
- 1 chocolate–hazelnut cream
- 1 ginger tea

During the afternoon
Green tea + spring water

Dinner
- Keto-pizza (see page 117)
- Rocket salad (with 1 tbsp of sacha inchi oil)
- 1 verbena tea

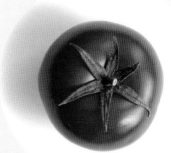
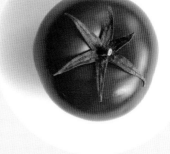

SUNDAY

On waking up Spring water

Breakfast
- Keto-adapted Budwig cream (2 tsp yogurt, coconut milk, 1 tbsp of sacha inchi oil, ½ lemon, 1 ground chia seeds and ½ tsp vanilla or cinnamon powder)
- 1 lemon and ginger herbal tea

Throughout the morning
Maté, herbal tea (rosemary, thyme or lemon and ginger) + spring water

Lunch
- 1 large glass of spring water
- Courgette spaghetti in tomato sauce with vegetable patties (see page 113)
- 1 square of 100 per cent dark chocolate or a few cacao beans
- 1 ginger tea

During the afternoon Green tea

Dinner
- Miso–sesame broth
- Sesame and miso black cream (see page 120), with raw vegetable sticks (cucumber or black radish)
- 1 chia seed yogurt with spices (see page 124)
- 1 anise or fennel tea

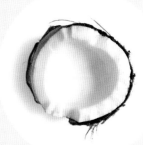

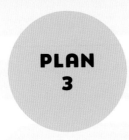

PLAN 3

THE VEGETARIAN & VEGAN PLAN

Contrary to popular belief, it's perfectly possible to be vegetarian or vegan and follow a balanced ketogenic diet.

There are certain things to watch out for, in particular a low intake of vitamin B_{12} and iron, and low levels of eicosapentaenoic acid (EPA) and docosahexaenoic acid (DHA), the active forms of omega-3s found mainly in oily fish. For vegans, focus on oily foods rich in fats and protein as well as raw foods. Also keep an eye on zinc and vitamin D intakes.

HOW TO FOLLOW THIS PLAN

- As with the other plans, begin with an intermittent fast of at least three days to enter into ketosis (first meal of the day at around 1 pm, last meal before 9 pm).
- Don't forget to be active and exercise regularly.
- Use test strips to check your state of ketosis every morning on an empty stomach. You'll see if you have slightly deviated straightaway. It's easy to come out of ketosis quickly.

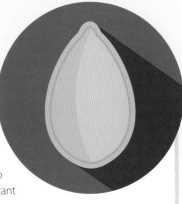

PLEASE NOTE!

- For vitamin B_{12}, you'll need to supplement with methylcobalamin, the active form of vitamin B_{12}. Opt for miso and certain algae. You'll also need to regularly measure your levels of cobalamin and homocysteine, very important markers that, when elevated, indicate deficiencies in B_9 and B_{12}.
- As for iron, particularly with women, it's important to always check your ferritin (iron storage), especially if your digestive tract isn't healthy, which may affect iron absorption – for example, if you have hypochlorhydria (low stomach acid) or inflammation of the intestinal lining. To make up for any shortfall, include spirulina flakes and rely on vitamin C (in acerola or camu camu, for example), which helps with the assimilation of plant irons. Also consider plants rich in iron, such as dulse seaweed, parsley, pumpkin seeds, spirulina, sesame puree, nettle leaf powder and raw cacao.
- For your EPA/DHA needs, vegetarians can eat two high-quality organic eggs and vegans seaweed tartare. If you don't want eggs, or simply to be on the safe side, supplement with EPA/DHA. Feel free to ask your doctor or naturopath for advice.

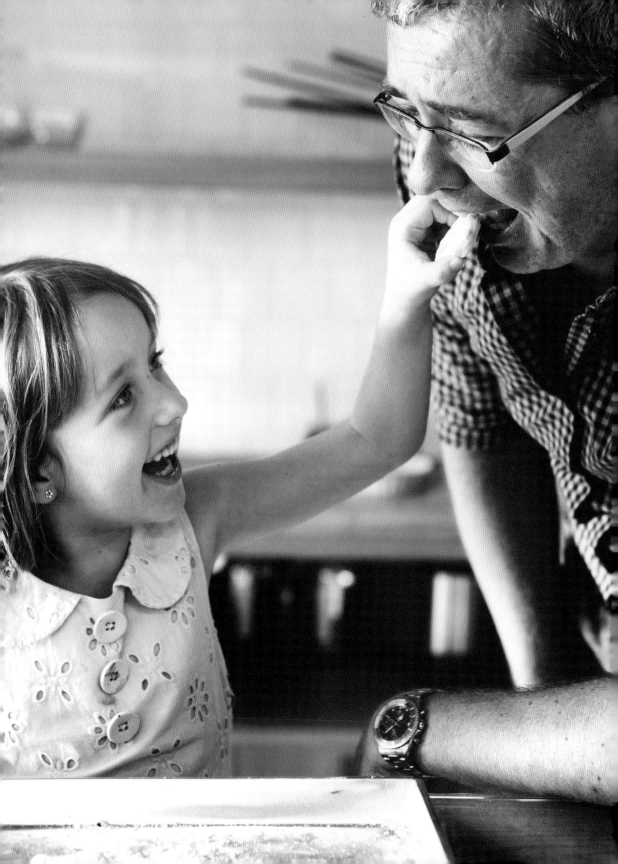

MENUS FOR THE WEEK

MONDAY

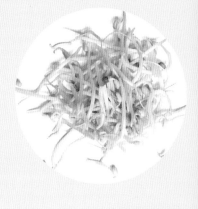

On waking up Spring water

Breakfast
- Almond porridge (almond milk, ground chia and flaxseeds,
  2 tbsp of hemp protein, almond flour and raw cacao – optional)
- 1 lemon and ginger herbal tea

Throughout the morning
Maté, herbal tea (rosemary, thyme or lemon and ginger) + spring water

Lunch
- 1 large glass of spring water
- For vegetarians: 2 poached eggs/sprouted seeds, baby spinach and olive salad
  (with 1 tbsp of camelina oil/sauerkraut crackers – see page 119)
- For vegans: macadamia nut hummus (see page 118) /1 avocado/sprouted seeds,
  baby spinach and seaweed flakes salad (with 1 tbsp of camelina oil and hemp seeds)
- 1 square of 100 per cent dark chocolate or a few cacao beans
- 1 ginger tea

During the afternoon Green tea, maté, herbal tea (rooibos, rosemary, thyme or hibiscus) + spring water

Dinner
- Gazpacho/avocado + 1 tsp of spirulina flakes/grated black radish salad
  (with 1 tsp of sacha inchi oil and hemp seeds)
- 1 cinnamon tea

TUESDAY

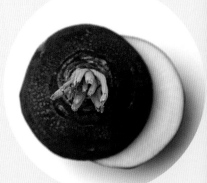

On waking up Spring water

Breakfast
- Sacha inchi smoothie (sacha inchi milk, ground chia seeds and flaxseeds,
  2 tbsp of hemp proteins, carob and vanilla)/maté + 1 tsp of coconut oil
- Rosemary or lemon thyme tea

Throughout the morning
Maté, herbal tea (rosemary, thyme or lemon and ginger) + spring water

Lunch
- 1 large glass of spring water
- Courgette-coconut pancakes (see page 116)/lacto-fermented vegetables/romaine salad (with 1 tbsp
  of camelina oil and shelled hemp seeds)/a few cacao beans + almonds
- 1 ginger or cinnamon tea

During the afternoon Green tea + spring water

Dinner
- Black radish salad + some sprouted lentils (with 1 tsp of sacha inchi oil and shelled hemp seeds)/
  steamed green asparagus/1 coconut milk yogurt + ½ tsp of vanilla powder
- 1 linden flower tea

WEDNESDAY

On waking up Spring water

Breakfast
- Chia seed porridge (almond milk, chia seeds, hemp proteins, vanilla and coconut cream)
- Rosemary tea

Throughout the morning
Maté, herbal tea (rosemary, thyme or lemon and ginger) + spring water

Lunch
- 1 large glass of spring water
- Leek and almond flour pancakes (see page 116)/lacto-fermented cucumbers, with 1 tbsp of camelina oil and hemp seeds/1 avocado
- 1 square of 100 per cent dark chocolate
- 1 ginger or rosemary tea

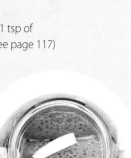

During the afternoon
Green tea, maté, herbal tea (rooibos, rosemary, thyme or hibiscus) + spring water

Dinner
- Grated black radish salad (with 1 tbsp of camelina oil and hemp seeds)/1 avocado + 1 tsp of spirulina flakes/steamed broccoli + coconut butter with fresh turmeric and ginger (see page 117)
- 1 lemon balm or cinnamon tea

THURSDAY

On waking up Spring water

Breakfast
- For vegetarians: 2 boiled eggs/1 avocado + 1 tsp of spirulina flakes
- For vegans: almond porridge (almond milk, ground chia seeds, 2 tbsp of pea protein, coconut cream and raw cacao – optional)
- Lemon and ginger herbal tea + 1 tsp coconut oil

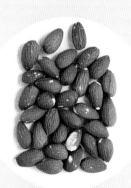

Throughout the morning
Maté, herbal tea (rosemary, thyme or lemon and ginger) + spring water

Lunch
- 1 large glass of spring water
- Macadamia nut cheese (see page 121)/endive salad (with 1 tsp of sacha inchi oil and walnut pieces)
- 1 square of 100 per cent dark chocolate or a few cacao beans
- 1 ginger or thyme tea

During the afternoon Green tea + spring water

Dinner
- Lacto-fermented vegetables
- Cauliflower tabbouleh
- Camomile tea + a few almonds

FRIDAY

On waking up Spring water

Breakfast
- Almond porridge (almond milk, ground chia seeds, rice protein, coconut cream and raw cacao – optional)
- Lemon and ginger herbal tea (+ 1 tsp coconut oil for vegans)

Throughout the morning
Maté, herbal tea (rosemary, thyme or lemon and ginger) + spring water

Lunch
- 1 large glass of spring water
- Guacamole/cashew nut flatbread (see page 110)/baby leaf, sprouted seeds and olive salad (with 1 tbsp of camelina oil)
- 1 square of 100 per cent dark chocolate or a few cacao beans
- 1 hibiscus or cinnamon tea

During the afternoon
Green tea + spring water

Dinner
- For vegetarians: kale salad (see page 109)/2 poached eggs
- For vegans: courgette spaghetti in tomato sauce with vegetable patties (see page 113)
- 1 coconut milk yogurt + 1 pinch of vanilla + 1 pinch of cinnamon
- 1 ginger or linden flower tea

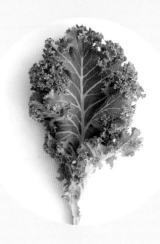

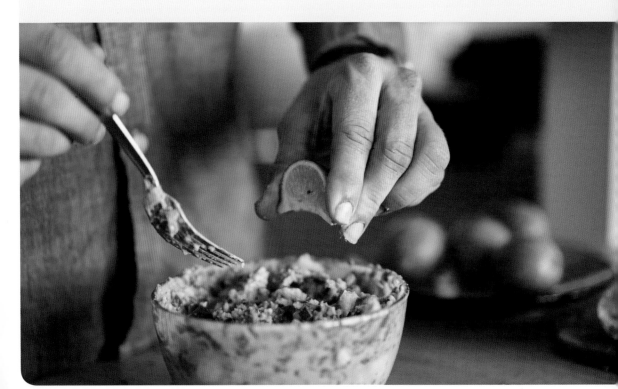

SATURDAY

On waking up Spring water

Breakfast
- For vegetarians: almond crepes (see page 122)/1 rosemary tea
- For vegans: avocado and almond milk–sesame smoothie/lemon and ginger herbal tea
  + 1 tsp coconut oil

Throughout the morning
Maté, herbal tea (rosemary, thyme or lemon and ginger) + spring water

Lunch
- 1 large glass of spring water
- For vegetarians: seaweed tartare (see page 119) + 1 avocado/runny omelette with mushrooms
  (2 eggs) + 1 tsp coconut oil for cooking/green salad (with 1 tsp of sacha inchi oil)
- For vegans: sprouted seeds, baby spinach, olive salad and other salad leaves, and macadamia
  cheese (with 1 tbsp of camelina oil, ground hemp seeds and flaxseeds)
- 1 square of 100 per cent dark chocolate or a few cacao beans
- 1 cinnamon or ginger tea

During the afternoon Maté + spring water

Dinner
- For vegetarians: cashew nut flatbread (see page 110), a few cacao beans + a few almonds
- For vegans: kale chips /keto-pizza (see page 117)
- 1 linden flower or verbena tea

SUNDAY

On waking up Spring water

Breakfast
- Cinnamon pancake (without eggs for vegans)
- Green tea + 1 tsp coconut oil

Throughout the morning
Maté, herbal tea (rosemary, thyme or lemon and ginger) + spring water

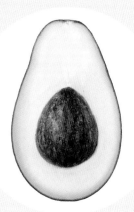

Lunch
- 1 large glass of spring water
- Lacto-fermented tofu with pesto
- 1 avocado
- Sprouted seeds, baby spinach, rocket and lamb's lettuce salad (with 1 tbsp of camelina oil
  and hemp seeds)
- Raw cacao brownie (see page 123)
- 1 ginger tea

During the afternoon Rooibos tea + spring water

Dinner
- Cooked cauliflower soup (see page 107)
- Sauerkraut crackers (see page 119)
- 1 verbena or lemon thyme tea

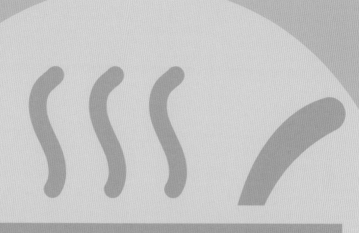

5
RECIPES

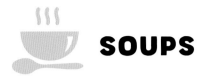

SOUPS

AVOCADO-CASHEW NUT SOUP
VEGETARIAN • VEGAN • GLUTEN FREE

Serves 4 • Preparation time: 10 minutes

Ingredients
4 ripe avocados
1 cucumber
2 handfuls of rocket
2 fresh small onions
2 lemons
1 pinch of Himalayan salt
Indian spices of your choice (such as powdered turmeric, cumin or ginger)

Method
• Cut open the avocados, remove the pits and scoop out the flesh. Peel the cucumber, remove the seeds and cut into large cubes. Rinse the rocket. Chop the small onions. Squeeze the juice from the lemons. Pour 400 ml (14 fl oz) of spring water into a blender, then add all the ingredients. Mix. Add the salt and spices of your choice. Serve immediately.

TIPS & VARIATIONS
• Just before serving, add fresh herbs of your choice (such as chives, fresh coriander or fresh mint), 1 tsp of coconut oil and 1 tsp of olive oil.

CREAMY SPINACH SOUP
VEGETARIAN • VEGAN • GLUTEN FREE

Serves 4 • Preparation time: 10 minutes

Ingredients
1 or 2 generous handfuls of fresh baby spinach
1 avocado
2 lemons
1 garlic clove
1 onion
1 tsp of dried rosemary
2 tbsp of pine nuts
3 tbsp of macadamia nuts

Method
• Rinse the baby spinach. Cut open the avocados, remove the pits and scoop out the flesh. Squeeze the juice from the lemons. Peel and roughly chop the garlic and the onion.
• Grind the pine nuts and macadamia nuts into a powder in a blender. Pour in 800 ml (27 fl oz) to 1 litre (2 pints) of spring water, add the remaining ingredients and mix in a blender to get a creamy texture.

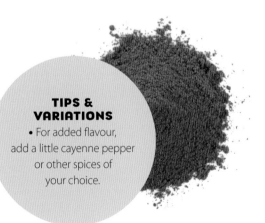

TIPS & VARIATIONS
• For added flavour, add a little cayenne pepper or other spices of your choice.

COOKED CAULIFLOWER SOUP
VEGETARIAN • VEGAN • GLUTEN FREE
Serves 4 • Preparation time: 15 minutes • Cooking time: 20 minutes

Ingredients
1 cauliflower
2 leeks
1 onion
2 cloves of garlic
4 tbsp of tahini (white sesame paste)
4 tbsp of coconut oil
1 pinch of Himalayan salt

Method
- Chop the cauliflower into small florets and rinse. Wash and slice the leeks. Peel and chop the onions and garlic.
- In a saucepan, melt the coconut oil over a gentle heat for 2 minutes. Add the leeks, cauliflower, onion and garlic. Cook on a gentle heat, while stirring, for 3–5 minutes.
- Pour in enough water to cover the ingredients, cover and cook for 10–15 minutes.
- Strain some of the soup over a saucepan to collect the broth. Mix it in a blender, then add as much broth as you need until you get the right consistency.
- Add the salt and tahini and blend again. Serve immediately.

SAVOY CABBAGE, LEEK & MISO SOUP
VEGETARIAN • VEGAN • GLUTEN FREE
Serves 4 • Preparation time: 10 minutes • Cooking time: 20 minutes

Ingredients
½ savoy cabbage
2 leeks
1 clove of garlic
2 pink peppercorns
1 juniper berry
1–2 tsp unpasteurized rice miso

Method
- Rinse and finely chop the cabbage. Wash and finely slice the leeks.
- In a large saucepan, pour in around 1 litre (2 pints) of spring water, then add all the ingredients. Cook over a medium heat for 20 minutes. Serve without blending.

TIPS & VARIATIONS
- Add a thinly sliced carrot or turnip.
- Vary the vegetables by season: green cabbage, courgettes, asparagus, spinach.
- To thicken the soup, add 1 tsp to 1 tbsp of psyllium or 1–2 tsp of ground chia seeds. Wait 10 minutes before tasting.

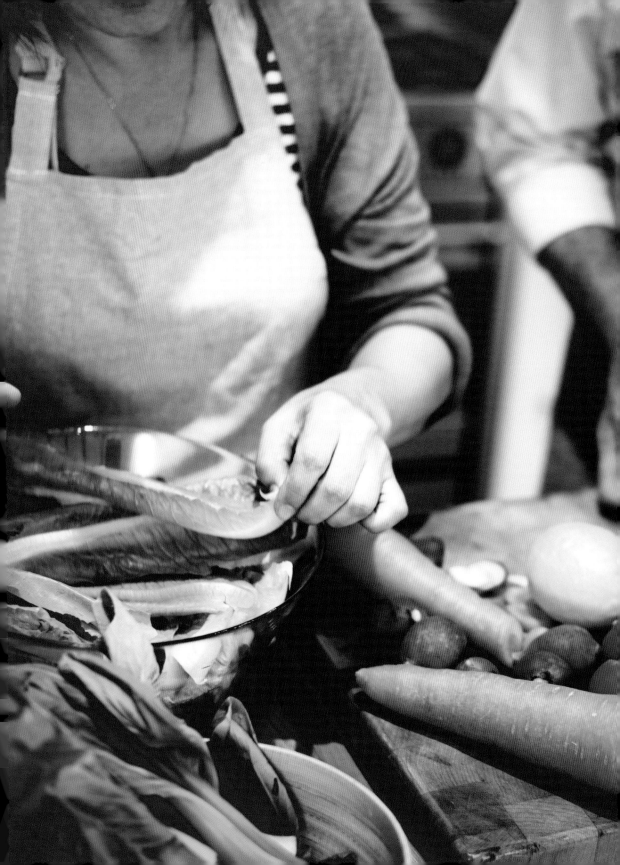

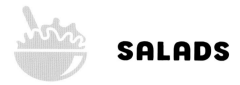

SALADS

SPROUTED SOY BEAN SALAD WITH PRAWNS & MACADAMIA NUTS

GLUTEN FREE

Serves 1 • Preparation time: 15 minutes • Waiting time: 1 hour

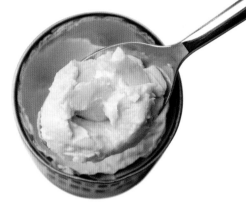

Ingredients

30 g (1 oz) of soy bean sprouts
¼ cucumber
6 cooked organic pink prawns
30 g (1 oz) of macadamia nuts
50 ml (1¾ fl oz) of coconut cream
½ tsp of curry powder
1 pinch of chilli powder
½ lime

Method

- Soak the macadamia nuts in spring water in a large bowl overnight.
- Rinse and drain the soy bean sprouts. Peel the cucumber and cut it into fine sticks.
- Roughly crush the drained macadamia nuts.
- In a bowl, mix the coconut cream with the juice of the lime, curry powder and chilli powder.
- Then mix the soy bean sprouts with the cucumber sticks, prawns and macadamia nuts. Pour the coconut–spice sauce over it, mix again and serve immediately.

KALE SALAD

VEGETARIAN • VEGAN • GLUTEN FREE

Serves 2 • Preparation time: 10 minutes

TIPS & VARIATIONS

- Massaging the kale leaves with the vinaigrette 'cooks' them. Do this for 10 minutes.
- For more colour in the salad, add small cherry tomatoes cut in two.

Ingredients

10 kale leaves
1 avocado
2 tbsp of tahini (white sesame paste)
1 tbsp of mustard
3 tbsp of sacha inchi or camelina oil
1 tbsp of ume plum vinegar
2 lemons

Method

- Wash and rinse the kale. Separate the leaves from the stalks in the middle and cut these into fine slices.
- In a bowl, mix the oil, vinegar, juice of 1 lemon, mustard and tahini to make a vinaigrette.
- Put the kale and vinaigrette into a salad bowl and massage the mixture well into the kale leaves.
- Cut the avocado into two. Remove the pit and cut the flesh into slices. Squeeze the juice of the second lemon over it. Add the avocado slices to the kale leaves. Mix again and serve immediately.

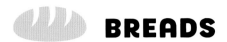 **BREADS**

CASHEW NUT FLATBREAD
VEGETARIAN • VEGAN • GLUTEN FREE

Makes 1 flat bread
Preparation time: 15 minutes • Waiting time: 1 night
• Cooking time: 4 hours

Ingredients
230 g (8 oz) of cashew nuts
80 g (2¾ oz) of blond psyllium powder
1 pinch of Himalayan salt
1 tsp of ground thyme or rosemary
1 small clove of garlic

Method
• Rehydrate and pre-sprout the cashew nuts overnight in a bowl of water.
• The next day, rinse and drain the cashew nuts. Peel and finely chop the garlic.
• Preheat the oven to 50°C (gas mark 1).
• Mix half the cashew nuts in a blender with 110 ml (4 fl oz) of spring water until you get a really smooth consistency. Add the garlic, the selected herb and salt. Mix again.
• Gradually add the psyllium, mixing it with 110 ml (4 fl oz) of spring water as well as the rest of the roughly chopped cashew nuts. Spread the mixture very thinly on a baking tray covered in parchment paper.
• Bake for around 4 hours. The bread should be dry. Cut into pieces and store in an airtight box.

TIPS & VARIATIONS
• Substitute the cashew nuts with macadamia nuts.
• Make this bread in a food dehydrator at 42°C (107°F), for around 5 hours – the bread should be crisp.
• Serve with guacamole, dips, raw vegetables or salads.

ALMOND FLOUR BREAD
VEGETARIAN • GLUTEN FREE

Makes 1 loaf
Preparation time: 10 minutes • Cooking time: 45 minutes

Ingredients
300 g (10½ oz) of low-carb almond flour
6 eggs
2 tbsp of coconut oil + 1 tbsp for greasing the tin
1 tsp of cider vinegar
½ tsp of sodium bicarbonate

Method
• Preheat the oven to 180°C (gas mark 6).
• Mix all the ingredients together, except the vinegar. Add the vinegar when the mixture is smoothly blended.
• Grease a loaf tin and pour in the dough. Bake for 40–45 minutes.

TIPS & VARIATIONS
• Substitute the almond flour with coconut flour, or make a mixture of the two flours. As the coconut flour is very high in fibre, you may need to add a little water to be able to mix the dough well.

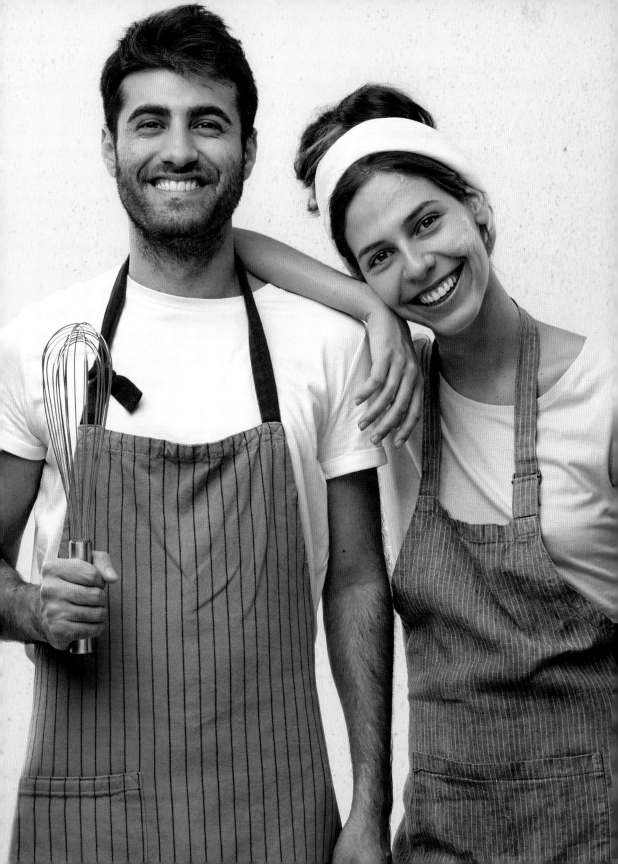

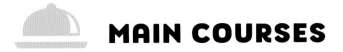

MAIN COURSES

COCONUT-ALMOND BREADED CHICKEN
GLUTEN FREE

Serves 1 • Preparation time: 10 minutes • Cooking time: 15 minutes

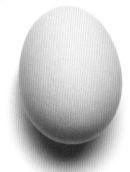

Ingredients

1 organic chicken breast
15 g (½ oz) of almond flour
20 g (¾ oz) of grated coconut
1 organic egg
1 tbsp of coconut oil
1 tsp of curry powder
Unrefined sea salt, freshly ground pepper

Method

- Crack the egg into a shallow bowl and whisk rapidly with a fork.
- In another shallow bowl, mix the almond powder, grated coconut, curry powder, salt and pepper.
- Dip the chicken breast in the beaten egg and soak it well. Then dip it into the almond–coconut powder mixture, to coat it completely.
- Heat the oil in a nonstick pan. Cook the chicken on a low heat for 10–15 minutes, turning it over regularly. Keep a close eye to prevent the chicken from burning as it cooks.

DUCK LEGS WITH OLIVES
GLUTEN FREE

Serves 4 • Preparation time: 10 minutes • Cooking time: 1.5 hours

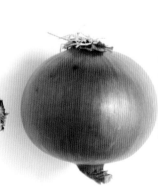

Ingredients

4 organic duck legs (120 g/4 oz of meat per person)
500 g (18 oz) of small button mushrooms
250 g (9 oz) of black olives
2 onions
1 sprig of rosemary
1 tbsp of duck fat
Unrefined sea salt, freshly ground pepper

Method

- Clean the mushrooms (leave them whole). Peel and finely slice the onions.
- Melt the duck fat in a casserole dish. Add the duck legs and brown them for 15 minutes on a low heat, turning from time to time.
- Add the mushroom, olives, sliced onions and rosemary sprig. Season with salt and pepper. Cover and cook on a low heat for 1 hour and 15 minutes.

COURGETTE SPAGHETTI IN TOMATO SAUCE WITH VEGETABLE PATTIES

VEGETARIAN • VEGAN • GLUTEN FREE

Serves 4 • Preparation time: 25 minutes • Cooking time: a few hours (patties)

Ingredients
For the spaghetti

5 courgettes

1 tbsp of lemon juice

1 tbsp of rapeseed or camelina oil

For the tomato sauce

6 sun-dried tomatoes

3 ripe tomatoes

12 lacto-fermented black olives

½ bunch of fresh basil

Oregano, spices of your choice (such as cumin, coriander or ginger)

For the vegetable patties

100 g (3½ oz) of macadamia nuts

3 tbsp of ground white chia seeds

1 garlic clove

1 tsp of unpasteurized rice miso

10 pitted black olives

3 tbsp of sacha inchi oil

2 tbsp of ume plum vinegar

½ tsp cumin

Fresh herbs of your choice (such as basil, marjoram, coriander or parsley)

Method

- Make the courgette spaghetti (you'll need a spiralizer).
- Make the tomato sauce: mix the ingredients together in a blender or food processor.
- Make the vegetable patties: mix the ingredients together in a food processor, then shape into small patties. Dehydrate these in a food dehydrator or in your oven for a few hours at 50°C (gas mark 1).
- Serve the spaghetti with the tomato sauce and patties.

TIPS & VARIATIONS

- You could also serve this spaghetti and patties with a salad of chopped raw button mushrooms mixed with lemon juice.

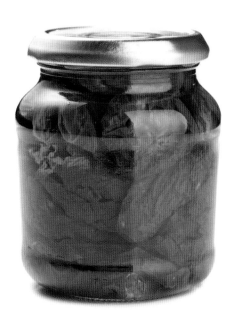

CAULIFLOWER RICE

VEGETARIAN • VEGAN • GLUTEN FREE

Serves 4 • Preparation time: 10 minutes • Cooking time: 7 minutes

Ingredients

1 cauliflower
2 tbsp of coconut oil
Unrefined sea salt, freshly ground pepper

Method

- Cut the cauliflower into small florets and rinse. Put them into the blender bowl and mix until it has the consistency of coarse semolina.
- Heat the coconut oil in a frying pan. Add the cauliflower rice, salt and pepper and cook for about 5–7 minutes on a medium heat, mixing regularly.

TIPS & VARIATIONS
- Flavour this rice with spices of your choice (such as cumin, curry powder, turmeric, ginger, coriander and cardamom).
- Substitute the coconut oil with red palm oil to give the dish a beautiful orange colour.

KALE SAUTÉED IN COCONUT OIL

VEGETARIAN • VEGAN • GLUTEN FREE

Serves 4 • Preparation time: 5 minutes • Cooking time: 12 minutes

Ingredients

16 kale leaves
2 tbsp of coconut oil
Spices of your choice (such as cumin, curry powder or ginger)

Method

- Wash the kale leaves, remove the central stalks and roughly chop the leaves. Steam-cook them for around 10 minutes.
- Melt the coconut oil in a saucepan over a low heat. Add the kale and spices. Cook on a medium heat for 1–2 minutes. Serve immediately.

CAULIFLOWER & COCONUT PUREE

VEGETARIAN • VEGAN • GLUTEN FREE

Serves 4 • Preparation time: 15 minutes • Cooking time: 15 minutes

Ingredients

1 cauliflower
150 ml (5 fl oz) of coconut cream
1 tbsp of coconut oil
½ tbsp of curry powder
Unrefined sea salt, freshly ground pepper

Method

- Cut the cauliflower into florets and rinse them. Steam-cook for 15 minutes.
- Mix the cauliflower with the coconut cream and coconut oil in a blender to get a smooth consistency. Add the curry powder, salt and pepper. Serve immediately.

BROCCOLI WITH COCONUT MILK, SESAME & SPICES

VEGETARIAN • VEGAN • GLUTEN FREE

Serves 4 • Preparation time: 5 minutes • Cooking time: 13 minutes

Ingredients

1 large broccoli
200 ml (7 fl oz) of coconut milk
1tsp of tahini (white sesame paste)
Spices of your choice (such as turmeric, cumin, coriander, ginger or paprika)

Method

• Cut the broccoli into florets, rinse and steam-cook for 8 minutes (they should remain slightly crisp).

• Pour the coconut milk, spices and tahini into a saucepan. Mix together and add the broccoli. Heat for 5 minutes on a low heat. Serve.

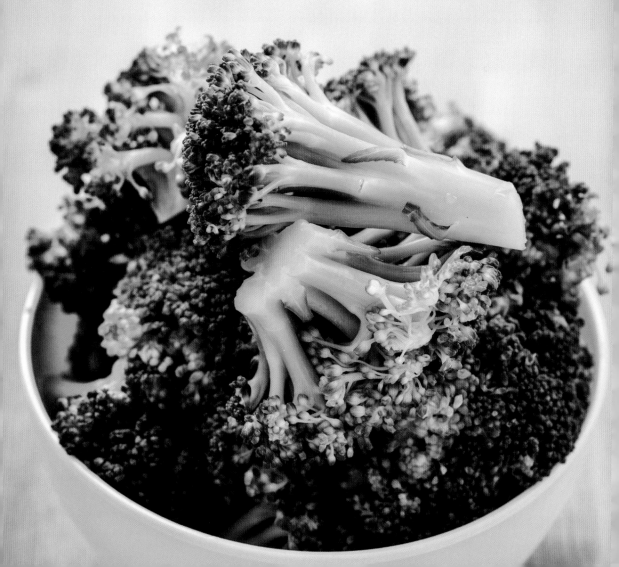

COURGETTE-COCONUT PANCAKES

VEGETARIAN • GLUTEN FREE

Makes around 10 pancakes
Preparation time: 15 minutes • Cooking time: 3–6 minutes per pancake

Ingredients

2 eggs
5 small courgettes
50 g (1¾ oz) of coconut flour
2 tbsp of coconut oil
Some fresh herbs (such as coriander or basil)
Spices of your choice (such as turmeric, cumin or coriander)
Unrefined sea salt

Method

- Wash and grate the courgettes. Rinse and finely chop the herbs.
- Beat the eggs with the flour, herbs, salt and spices. Add the grated courgettes and mix.
- Heat a splash of oil in the pan. Pour a little of the mixture into the pan and cook the pancakes for 3–6 minutes on each side (depending on their thickness). Serve hot.

TIPS & VARIATIONS

- Substitute the coconut flour with organic low-carb almond flour.
- Substitute the courgettes with small leeks (cook them a few minutes beforehand) or grated cabbage.

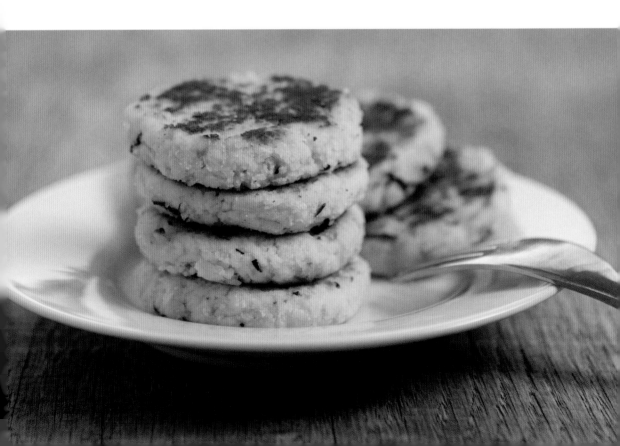

KETO-PIZZA WITH SEEDS

VEGETARIAN • VEGAN • GLUTEN FREE

Serves 4 • Preparation time: 25 minutes • Waiting time: a few hours

Ingredients

150 g (5 oz) of activated sunflower seeds
150 g (5 oz) of ground flaxseeds
2 tbsp of sacha inchi oil
6 pitted black olives
1 garlic clove
Fresh herbs (such as oregano, basil, thyme, marjoram or rosemary)
1 pinch of salt

Method

- Pour all the ingredients into a blender and mix until you get a fairly fine flour.
  Add 200–350 ml (7–12 fl oz) of water to make a malleable dough, neither too dry nor too wet.
- Spread the dough onto parchment paper and make a pizza shape.
- Let the pizza stand in the refrigerator for a few hours.
- Examples of a pizza topping could be: homemade fresh tomato sauce (blend together 2 very ripe fresh tomatoes + 5 dried tomatoes rehydrated in rapeseed oil + 1 garlic clove + a few fresh basil leaves + the juice of 1 lemon + 1 pinch of salt), macadamia nut cheese (see page 121), black olives and fresh herbs (such as basil, rocket or baby leaves).

COCONUT BUTTER WITH FRESH TURMERIC & GINGER

VEGETARIAN • VEGAN • GLUTEN FREE

Preparation time: 5 minutes

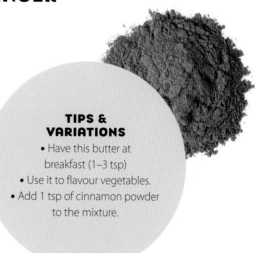

Ingredients

6 organic fresh turmeric roots
1 cm (½ in) of organic fresh ginger
4–5 tbsp of coconut oil

Method

- Thinly peel the turmeric and ginger.
- Mix together in a powerful food processer with 4–5 tbsp of coconut oil.
- Pour into a glass jar and store in a cool place. This butter will keep for 1 week.

TIPS & VARIATIONS

- Have this butter at breakfast (1–3 tsp)
- Use it to flavour vegetables.
- Add 1 tsp of cinnamon powder to the mixture.

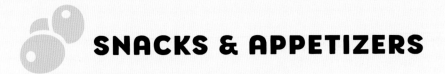

SNACKS & APPETIZERS

MACADAMIA NUT HUMMUS
VEGETARIAN • VEGAN • GLUTEN FREE

Serves 4 • Preparation time: 10 minutes • Waiting time: overnight

Ingredients

70 g (2½ oz) of macadamia nuts
1 garlic clove
2 tbsp of tahini (white sesame paste)
2 tbsp of sacha inchi oil
1 lemon
½ tsp of pasteurized rice miso
A few fresh basil leaves

Method

- Soak the macadamia nuts overnight in a bowl of spring water.
- The following day, peel and roughly chop the garlic. Squeeze the juice from the lemon. Rinse and finely chop the basil.
- Drain and rinse the nuts, then mix them in a blender. Add the garlic, sesame paste, sacha inchi oil, lemon juice and miso. Add the basil and serve with vegetable sticks.

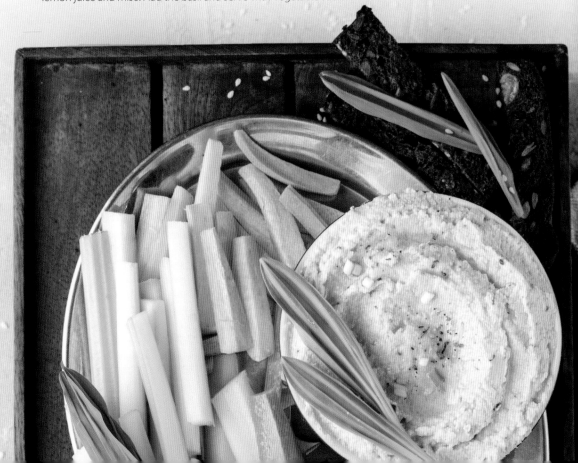

FRESH SEAWEED TARTARE
VEGETARIAN • VEGAN • GLUTEN FREE

Serves 4 • Preparation time: 20 minutes • Waiting time: a few hours or overnight

Ingredients
250 g (9 oz) of organic fresh sea lettuce
1 garlic clove
2 small shallots
15 black olives
6 capers
2 tbsp of camelina or sacha inchi oil
2 tbsp of olive oil
1 tbsp of ume plum vinegar

TIPS & VARIATIONS
• Substitute the black olives with olive tartare.
• Serve your tartare on avocado slices.

Method
• Soak the sea lettuce in a large bowl of spring water for 2 minutes.
• Drain by pressing it between your hands to remove as much water and salt as possible.
• Repeat once more.
• Spread the seaweed on a cutting board and cut into thin slices.
• Peel and chop the garlic and shallots. Finely chop the black olives and capers.
• In a salad bowl, mix the seaweed, garlic, shallots, olives and capers. Add the oils and vinegar and leave it to marinate for several hours or overnight.

SAUERKRAUT CRACKERS
VEGETARIAN • VEGAN • GLUTEN FREE

Makes about 20 crackers
Preparation time: 15 minutes • Waiting time: overnight • Cooking time: 1.5 hours

Ingredients
200 g (7 oz) raw sauerkraut
90 g (3 oz) of almonds
30 g (1 oz) of brazil nuts
90 g (3 oz) of sunflower seeds
3 tbsp of olive oil
1 tbsp of tahini (white sesame paste)
1 tbsp of tamari or 1 tbsp of unpasteurized rice miso
1 pinch of Himalayan salt

Method
• Rehydrate the almonds, brazil nuts and sunflower seeds in three separate bowls of spring water overnight.
• The following day, preheat the oven to 110°C (gas mark 3).
• Mix the seeds separately in a blender. Then add them to the rest of the ingredients in a salad bowl. Mix until you get a firm dough.
• Pour the mixture onto a baking tray covered in parchment paper. Flatten the mixture, using a spatula, to make a large crepe, keeping it thin and compact.
• Cook for 1.5 hours until the dough is crisp. Cut into crackers and store in an airtight container.

SESAME & MISO BLACK CREAM

VEGETARIAN • VEGAN • GLUTEN FREE

Makes 1 small bowl • Preparation time: 5 minutes

Ingredients

1 tbsp of black sesame paste
1 tbsp of almond puree
1 tsp of unpasteurized rice miso
1 tbsp of olive oil
1 tbsp of camelina oil
1 tsp of mustard

Method

• Pour all the ingredients into a bowl and mix together.

TIPS & VARIATIONS

• Eat with a raw salad, as a dip or with sticks of radish, cucumber, endives and celery.
• Turn this cream into a sauce by adding another 2 tbsp of oil (1 tbsp olive oil + 1 tbsp camelina oil, for example). In this case, change the measurement for the oily items from tbsp to tsp.

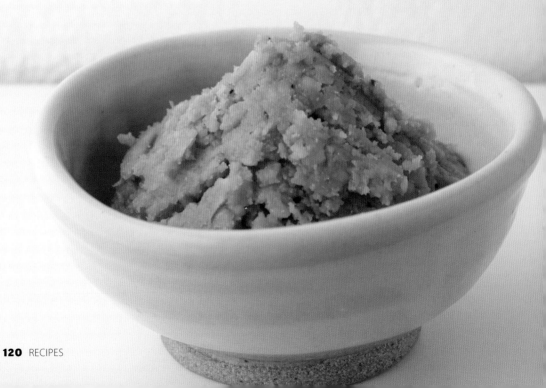

AVOCADO PESTO WITH ACAI
VEGETARIAN • VEGAN • GLUTEN FREE

Serves 4 • Preparation time: 5 minutes

Ingredients
1 ripe avocado
1 tsp of acai
1 tbsp of tahini
½–1 tsp of unpasteurized rice miso
½ lemon
1 tsp of sacha inchi oil

Method
• Cut open the avocado, remove the pit and scoop out the flesh. Squeeze the juice from the lemon.
• Mix all the ingredients together in a blender. Serve immediately.

MACADAMIA NUT CHEESE
VEGETARIAN • VEGAN • GLUTEN FREE

Makes about 300 g (10½ oz) of cheese • Preparation time: 10 minutes
• Waiting time: 12–24 hours

Ingredients
300 g (10½ oz) of macadamia nuts
1 tbsp of unrefined salt (fleur de sel or Guérande salt)
2 garlic cloves
A few sprigs of fresh chives
½ tsp of cumin (optional)

Method
• Pour the nuts and salt into a salad bowl. Cover with spring water and put a plate over the bowl. Leave to soak at room temperature for 12–24 hours.
• The following day, drain the nuts and mix them in a blender. Add the rinsed and chopped chives, peeled garlic clove and the cumin (if wanted). Mix again in the blender.
• Pour the mixture into a plant-milk bag (a cloth bag for filtering plant juice, sold in specialist shops) and squeeze to remove as much water as possible.
• Pour the mixture into a glass jar. This cheese can be stored in a cool place for three days.

TIPS & VARIATIONS
• Serve with avocados, vegetables or toast made with oily breads.
• Try replacing the cumin with basil or tarragon.

DESSERTS & PLANT MILKS

ALMOND CREPES
VEGETARIAN • GLUTEN FREE

Makes about 20 crepes • Preparation time: 5 minutes • Cooking time: 1 minute per crepe

Ingredients
4 eggs
200 g (7 oz) of white almond puree
2 tbsp of coconut oil
1 pinch of salt

Method
- In a blender, or by hand, mix the eggs, almond puree, 200 ml (7 fl oz) of water, 1 tbsp of coconut oil and the salt.
- Melt a little coconut oil in a pan. Pour in a ladleful of dough and cook the crepe for 30 seconds on each side. Cook the remaining crepes in the same way.

AVOCADO-CACAO MOUSSE
VEGETARIAN • VEGAN • GLUTEN FREE

Serves 2 • Preparation time: 10 minutes

Ingredients
2 ripe avocados
3 tbsp of cocoa butter
20 g (¾ oz) of raw cacao powder
2 tbsp of raw cacao nibs
1 tsp of raw carob powder
2 vanilla pods
2 tsp of cinnamon

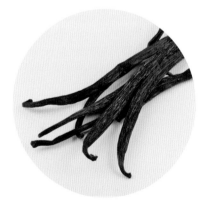

Method
- Melt the cocoa butter in a saucepan over a low heat. Let it cool and then add the carob.
- Cut open the avocados, remove the pits and scoop out the flesh.
- In a blender, mix the avocado flesh with the cacao powder, vanilla, cinnamon and cacao nibs, until you get a smooth and even texture. Add the cocoa butter to the carob.
- Pour into two small ramekins and serve.

RAW CACAO BROWNIES

VEGETARIAN • VEGAN • GLUTEN FREE

Serves 4 • Preparation time: 15 minutes • Cooking time: 20 minutes

Ingredients

100 g (3½ oz) of pecan nuts
60 ml (2 fl oz) of almond milk
40 g (1½ oz) of almond flour
4 tbsp of cacao powder
2 vanilla pods
1 tsp of cinnamon
2 tbsp of pea proteins
1 tbsp of melted cocoa butter + a little more to grease the baking tin
1 pinch of stevia

Method

- Split the vanilla pods and scoop out the small black seeds, using the tip of a knife.
- Preheat the oven to 180°C (gas mark 6).
- In a food processor, grind the pecan nuts to a coarse powder. Add the warmed almond milk, stevia, almond flour, cacao, vanilla, cinnamon and pea protein to make a smooth and even dough. Mix again in the food processor.
- When the mixture is nice and smooth, pour it in the mould greased with cocoa butter. Cook for 20 minutes.

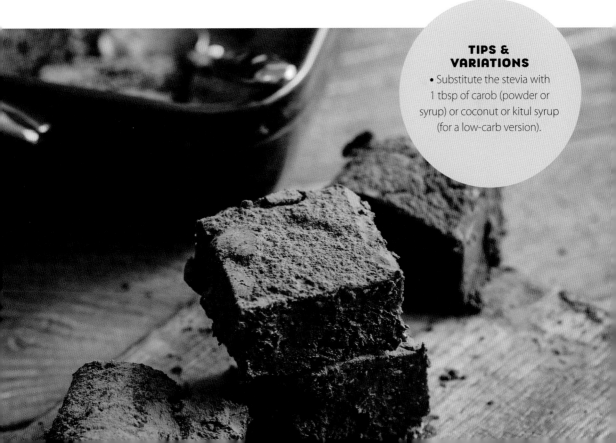

TIPS & VARIATIONS
- Substitute the stevia with 1 tbsp of carob (powder or syrup) or coconut or kitul syrup (for a low-carb version).

CHIA SEED YOGURT WITH SPICES

VEGETARIAN • VEGAN • GLUTEN FREE

Serves 2 • Preparation time: 5 minutes • Waiting time: 10 minutes + 4 hours

Ingredients

3 tbsp of ground chia seeds

400 ml (14 fl oz) of almond milk, sacha inchi milk (homemade, if possible, see below) or coconut milk

1 tsp of vanilla powder

1 tsp of cinnamon powder

Method

- In a salad bowl, mix together the ground chia seeds, plant milk and spices. Let the mixture stand for 10 minutes, then mix again. If the texture is too firm for your taste, add a little plant milk and mix once more.
- Let it stand for at least 4 hours in a cool place before serving. This yogurt can be stored for up to three days in a fridge.

TIPS & VARIATIONS

- Add blueberries or raspberries, depending on the level of carbohydrates you wish to consume during the day.
- Substitute the vanilla and cinnamon with 2 tsp of acai.
- For a chia seed yogurt with cacao: 3 tbsp chia seeds + 400 ml (14 fl oz) of coconut milk + 3 tbsp of melted cocoa butter + 1 tbsp of raw cacao powder and + 1 tbsp of cacao nibs.

PLANT MILKS

VEGETARIAN • VEGAN • GLUTEN FREE

You can make many plant milks yourself …

- Vanilla almond milk: 1 cup of almonds + 1 vanilla pod + 1 litre (4 cups/2 pints) of spring water (plus extra, for rehydrating). Soak the almonds in water for at least 8 hours or overnight. Rinse, then blend with the spring water for at least 1 minute. Strain the mixture, using a nut milk bag or thin dish towel. Add the seeds from the vanilla pod to the strained liquid, then blend for another 30 seconds. Pour the milk into a glass bottle and store in a cool place.

In the same way

- Vanilla macadamia milk: 1 cup of macadamia nuts to rehydrate + 1 vanilla pod + 1 litre (4 cups/2 pints) of spring water + 2 pitted and rehydrated dates (optional, for a low-carb version).
- Vanilla hemp milk: 50 g (1¾ oz) of hemp seeds + 1 vanilla pod + 1 litre (4 cups/2 pints) of spring water + 2 pitted and rehydrated dates (optional, for a low-carb version).
- Sacha inchi and hazelnut milk: 15–20 sacha inchi seeds to rehydrate + 1 vanilla pod + 1 litre (4 cups/2 pints) of spring water + 1 tsp of hazelnut puree + 2 pitted and rehydrated dates (optional, for a low-carb version).

GOLDEN TURMERIC MILK

VEGETARIAN • VEGAN • GLUTEN FREE

Serves 1 • Preparation time: 5 minutes • Cooking time: 5 minutes

Ingredients

200 ml (7 fl oz) coconut milk
1 tsp of homemade coconut butter with turmeric (see page 117)
1 tsp of coconut oil

Method

• Pour all the ingredients in a saucepan and mix.
• Heat on a very low heat for 5 minutes.

**TIPS &
VARIATIONS**
• You can add ½ tsp of
cinnamon, or a little kitul
or coconut syrup (for a
low-carb version).

INDEX

PICTURE CREDITS

Front Cover Moremar/ShutterStockphoto.Inc

ShutterStockphoto.Inc 1 Moremar; 2 Graf Vishenka; 3 Moremar; 6 Foxys Forest Manufacture; 12 Graf Vishenka; 13 Foxys Forest Manufacture; 15 Rawpixel.com; 16, 19 StudioPhotoDFlorez; 20 Jiri Hera; 21 Josep Suria; 23 Vorontsova Anastasiia; 25 Anna de la Cruz; 26 Daxiao Productions; 29 Jacob Lund; 30, 31 Uniyok; 32 Y Photo Studio; 33 SofiaV; 34 StudioPhotoDFlorez; 35 Viktoria Yams; 37 t cr StudioPhotoDFlorez; 37 cl Oko Laa, 37 b Anatolir; 38 Viktor1; 39 successo images; 40 Anatolir; 41 Viktorija Reuta; 42, 43 StudioPhotoDFlorez; 44 SofiaV; 45 Rawpixel.com; 46 RedlineVector; 47 StudioPhotoDFlorez; 48 Suto Norbert Zsolt; 49 t b, 50, 51 StudioPhotoDFlorez; 52 Anatolir; 53 StudioPhotoDFlorez; 55 Tanya Sid; 56 Africa Studio; 57 kazoka; 58 Africa Studio; 60 Vorontsova Anastasiia; 63 Ganihina Daria; 67 shapovalphoto; 68 BarracudaDesigns; 69 Rawpixel.com; 70 zoryanchik; 74 Foxys Forest Manufacture; 76 Inna Zueva Nikolaevna; 79 Rawpixel.com; 86 VGstockstudio; 87 Yury Velikanov; 88 Gayvoronskaya_Yana; 89, 90 t c Studio PhotoDFlorez; 90 b Bozena Fulawka; 91 t StudioPhotoDFlorez; 91 b Jiri Hera; 93 t StudioPhoto DFlorez; 93 b Daryna Khozieieva; 94 t Coprid; 94 c b, 95 t StudioPhotoDFlorez; 95 b Brent Hofacker; 96 t StudioPhotoDFlorez; 96 b Martin Rettenberger; 97 StudioPhotoDFlorez; 98 Rvector; 99 Rawpixel. com; 100 t StudioPhotoDFlorez; 100 b Markus Jaaske; 101 t Marina Shanti; 101 c Aleksandra Duda; 101 b, 102 t StudioPhotoDFlorez; 102 b Joshua Resnick; 103 Moving Moment; 106 SOMMAI; 107 tim08; 108 Rawpixel.com; 109 t Africa Studio; 109 b StudioPhotoDFlorez; 111 WAYHOME studio; 112 t Bozena Fulawka; 112 b StudioPhotoDFlorez; 113 Jiri Hera; 115 gephoto; 116 Lilly Trott; 117 t Rtstudio; 117 b Matyi012345; 118 Tukhfatullina Anna; 119 StudioPhotoDFlorez; 120 ITO_IKI; 122 GoncharukMaks; 123 July Prokopiv; 125 MasterQ

Graphic artworks The Noun Project (thenounproject.com)

ACKNOWLEDGEMENTS

Eddison Books Limited
Managing Director Lisa Dyer
Creative Consultant Nick Eddison
Managing Editor Tessa Monina
Translation Lalit Nadkarni
Designed and edited by Fogdog Creative (www.fogdog.co.uk)
Proofreader Jane Roe
Indexer Marie Lorimer
Production Sarah Rooney & Cara Clapham